AIDS Treatment and Human Rights in Context

Also by Peris S. Jones:

Democratising Development: The Politics of Socio-Economic Rights in South Africa, co-edited with K. Stokke, 2005

AIDS Treatment and Human Rights in Context

Peris S. Jones

palgrave
macmillan

AIDS TREATMENT AND HUMAN RIGHTS IN CONTEXT

First published in 2009 by PALGRAVE MACMILLAN® in the United States—a division of St. Martin's Press LLC, 175 Fifth Avenue, New York, NY 10010.

Where this book is distributed in the UK, Europe, and the rest of the world, this is by Palgrave Macmillan, a division of Macmillan Publishers Limited, registered in England, company number 785998, of Houndmills, Basingstoke, Hampshire RG21 6XS.

Palgrave Macmillan is the global academic imprint of the above companies and has companies and representatives throughout the world.

Palgrave® and Macmillan® are registered trademarks in the United States, the United Kingdom, Europe and other countries.

ISBN-13: 978-0-230-60959-4
ISBN-10: 0-230-60959-7

Library of Congress Cataloging-in-Publication Data is available from the Library of Congress.

A catalogue record of the book is available from the British Library.

Design by Scribe Inc.

First edition: May 2009.

10 9 8 7 6 5 4 3 2 1

Printed in the United States of America.

Peris Jones, "A test of Governance": Rights-based struggles and the politics of HIV/AIDS policy in South Africa, *Political Geography* 2005; 24(4):419–47, from which several pages are adapted in Chapter 1 and Chapter 2.

Table 2.1 is based upon Peris Jones, "On a never ending waiting list": Towards equitable access to antiretroviral treatment? Experiences from Zambia. *Health and Human Rights*, special issue on HIV/AIDS, 8, 2, (December).

To Astrid, Anja, and Ellie, the brightest,
most dazzling of lights in my life

Contents

Foreword

The N1 highway darts northwards from Pretoria, straight as an arrow through flat open *bushveld*. The road is in pristine condition. It deceives. Occasionally adorned by service stations replete with snack bars and verdant green lawns complemented by equally lush fountains gushing water, the contrast awaiting could not have been starker. Taking the Hammanskraal highway "off-ramp" for the first time was a stark reminder of those many parts of South Africa shaped by forced settlement and, where, amongst the brickmaking workshops and roadside car exhausts sales, severe material challenges infuse daily life. But not far from the local hospital, *Jubilee*, a corrugated tin shack daubed with the word "Herbalist," announces also other challenges to do with competing notions of health and illness (see Fig. 0.1; Herbalist, Hammanskraal, and all other photos, A. Murray). All this, out of sight, and I daresay, out of mind for most inhabitants of the minority verdant green world paying their N1 highway toll. This is how the study began: a morning coffee in such a service station, and by afternoon, the first stack of a series of stories reflecting death, exclusion, confusion, and competing beliefs—all in an era when AIDS medication was denied to South Africans in the public health system. By 2005, with the era of antiretroviral treatment finally underway at *Jubilee*, all this was to change, wasn't it?

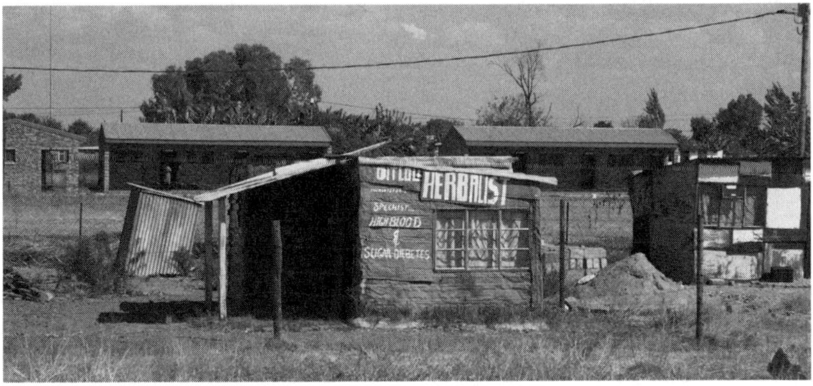

Figure 0.1 Herbalist, Hammanskraal

Acknowledgments

The genesis of the book, as with most creative work, took place long before any writing or conscious conceptualization ever did. While it has built on layers of experience accumulated over the years, my work on AIDS only started in 2002. And, rather self-conscious as I was about being another addition to this massive and congested field of enquiry and practice, four particular moments all provided much needed solidity for my subsequent attempts to understand and experience the epidemic.

In a seminar in Oslo in 2002, commenting on a United Nations Development Program (UNDP) presentation, upon apologizing for my "newness" in working on AIDS, the UNDP staff member in question responded along the lines of, "do not apologize, the sector needs people with fresh thoughts, unencumbered by the prevailing wisdom." This had deep resonance for me, for which I thank the presenter, Lee-Nah Hsu. Then, my particular "moment of truth" concerning AIDS in South Africa really came thanks to the Community Law and Rural Development Centre (CLRDC) to whom I owe a great debt. Once upon a time, the CLRDC had an impressive network of paralegal offices working in some of the poorest and most rural parts of KwaZulu Natal. These offices, amongst other things, provided legal support to communities and clawed back an impressive amount of income from social grant entitlements and other untapped sources. In 2003, the CLRDC was kind enough to host me for some months in Durban. The latter visit included accompanying Irene Chetty and Sandile Sithole on one of their field visits to several of the paralegal offices across the province. Afterwards, I was lucky enough to be hooked up in Hluhluwe with the CLRDC's Langa Mtshali. By then I thought I was beginning to acquire a little knowledge about AIDS. But it was not until I accompanied one of the CLRDC's paralegals and a social worker making some home visits to people living with AIDS in a location in Hluhluwe, however, that upon seeing the ravages of the disease in the intimacy of family life and home settings, had I learnt anything by way of comparison. In an era when the location was served only by a mobile clinic and ARVs were still unavailable in the public sector, the experiences witnessed behind closed doors, in such close proximity to the gentle beauty of the green rolling hills of the Hluhluwe game reserve and the bus loads of affluent tourists disembarking there, was both profoundly moving and disturbing.

It was also around this time, many years after I first knew of him in Gaborone, Botswana, that I was therefore fortunate to be reacquainted with Mark Heywood of the AIDS Law Project and Treatment Action Campaign. At the height of the South African government's efforts to block the roll out of antiretrovirals (ARVs), Mark very kindly agreed to fly to Oslo to do a presentation at the Norwegian Centre for Human Rights. Meeting Mark then and since, and in reading his written work, has all been immensely influential in seeking to envisage ways to bring much needed animation to otherwise sterile debates on health and human rights. Indeed, Mark has provided the sharpest of intellectual knives for both South African and global AIDS activists to cut through the denials and barriers in access to ARVs. Mark's consistent focus, dedication, and generosity in giving people his time when the demands upon him are overwhelming have all been deeply inspirational.

In 2004, the South Africa Programme at the Norwegian Centre for Human Rights began collaboration with the Centre for the Study of AIDS (CSA), University of Pretoria, on the Hammanskraal-based *Tswelopele* project. It was very fortuitous timing to be involved in the development of such an exciting project, and one blessed by its very able project manger, Farhana Zuberi. I thank her for our fruitful collaboration that laid some of the foundations for the book. In 2006 to mid-2007, the CSA very kindly hosted me as a visiting postdoctoral fellow for a year and a half. I owe a massive debt of gratitude to CSA for being the best of hosts, and above all, in providing such a stimulating work environment. Jimmy Pieterse gets a particular mention for all those lively discussions, and also Johan Maritz, not least for both showing me another meaning of *Aand-Klas*. Rakgadi Mohlahlane was another important source for many stimulating moments of academic and social conversation. Two particular members of CSA deserve special acknowledgement. Pierre Brouard provided endless quantities of support for the project and a wicked sense of humor, particularly at a time when the research was floundering. Pierre's continuous dedication to his work on AIDS remains another great source of inspiration. Solomon Shirinda, previously office manager at the CSA's satellite office in Hammanskraal, also deserves special mention. It was not only Solly's fundamental role and patience in facilitating the fieldwork for which I am grateful to him and CSA. But in driving around Hammanskraal, even on the hottest and most parched of days, the obvious enjoyment Solly brought to community-level work meant, nonetheless, it was simply a pleasure to be with him.

Also at the University of Pretoria, at the Centre for Human Rights, I would like to thank both Frans Viljoen and Danie Brand for many inspiring conversations concerning human rights in South Africa, and across the continent. The anthropologist Saakie Niehaus (now at Brunel University) provided lunch hours filled with challenging discussion. Another debt is owed to the Department of Sociology, particularly Kamilla Naidoo, for hosting presentations of my work on two occasions in the exciting environment that Department has created. I am very grateful for the opportunity given to develop this and associated work, particularly at a time when these topics were so visibly such a fraught area of discussion.

Susan Craddock at the University of Minnesota was incredibly generous in providing time to look through an earlier version of the manuscript. This feedback helped immensely in developing it into a final book. Thank you for taking the time, Susan. Also in the States, Elizabeth Skeen, and her father, were immensely kind in copying and posting me a full copy of the Zuma rape case transcript. Their assistance is warmly acknowledged. Matthew Splitek, who was an intern at the Centre for the Study of AIDS in 2006, assisted in writing the section on South Africa and WHO's treatment guidelines.

And none of this would have been possible without the very generous support and freedom given to me by my previous employer, the South Africa Programme at the Norwegian Centre for Human Rights. I greatly acknowledge many of my colleagues there who, in one way or another, helped to facilitate my work on South Africa, these include: Kristin Høgdahl, Siri Skåre, Charlotte Norby, and her successor, Tor Kjetil Edland, and Bård Anders Andreassen, amongst others. The good working cooperation between the South Africa Programme and the Royal Norwegian Embassy in Pretoria is also greatly acknowledged, not least with Inger Stolle, Håkon Gulbrandsen, and also many good discussions with Thomas Ball, amongst others. I would also like to acknowledge the Network on Contextual Politics in Developing Countries based at the University of Oslo and who provided a small grant to cover some field work costs in South Africa. In particular, Kristian Stokke, Professor in Human Geography at the University of Oslo has provided valuable support over the years, both through this network but also far beyond it.

And many South African partners of the South Africa Programme have, through cooperation with the Programme, provided a very learned and colourful milieu that has been immensely beneficial in my attempts to understand human rights in South Africa and the region. In addition to the work of CSA, I should therefore also mention in particular the dynamism of Jackie Dugard and Stuart Wilson at the Centre for Applied Legal Studies at the University of Witswatersrand; and also Sibonile Khoza, who was previously manager of the

Socio-Economic Rights Project at the University of the Western Cape. Also, on two very special occasions, in 2004 in Oslo and then in 2008 at the University of London, I have been lucky enough to have invited Albie Sachs to give what can only be described as truly wonderful and inspirational speeches that continue to resonate. Between 2007 and 2008, I lectured for a year on a Masters course in human rights at the Institute of Commonwealth Studies, University of London. Although this book was written during my time at the Norwegian Centre for Human Rights, some fine-tuning of the ideas resulted from interaction with students in London.

Many thanks also to Alan Murray for providing the illustrations and, not least, many great moments when he visited South Africa in April 2007. Thanks also to all involved at Palgrave Macmillan, and also Danny Constantino at Scribe for such a smooth production process. Finally, this book would not have been finished had it not been for my remarkable partner, Astrid. Your unwavering support throughout the roller-coaster process and immense role in finalizing the book is deeply appreciated. But beyond this rock of support and your tolerance (pushed to the brink, it has to be said!) amidst my academic obsessing, it is your endless capacity for incisive and intelligent observation that amazes me even more. The biggest debt of all goes to you. Thank you so much.

Any mistakes or omissions, however, remain mine, and mine, alone.

Oslo, December 2008

Illustrations

Tables

Figures

Introduction

In terms of global access to AIDS treatment, the world has witnessed a seismic shift, and one in which human rights played such a catalytic role. In 2001, for sub-Saharan Africa in particular, whereas the figure once stood at 50,000, by the end of 2007, approximately 2 million people were able to access antiretroviral medication (ARVs).[1] Coverage now stands at approximately 30 percent of those who would benefit from access (WHO 2008). While falling well short of universal access, in light of the earlier, appalling paucity of access to ARVs, it is a dramatic increase nonetheless. From occupying a marginal position in global policy and conscience, AIDS treatment became mainstreamed in both policy debates and popular responses. Fêted by leaders and celebrities, and, through the Nelson Mandela *46664* campaign, capable of mobilizing thousands to attend pop concerts, AIDS treatment became cool. Human rights inspired political action, activism, and global declarations and funding commitments, all of which added a critical mass to the momentum in expanding access. Indeed, the struggle for AIDS treatment has been associated with enhancing political liberalization and liberal public health approaches (de Waal 2006). It may appear strange, then, to suggest that the "treatment era" is now possibly not turning out to be quite as reciprocal to human rights as the latter has been to struggles to get ARVs. Increasingly, this era is one that is becoming replete with a number of paradoxes that have harmful implications for both treatment programs and human rights. This book looks at these paradoxes as well as the undoubted benefits of ARVs.

The overarching paradox is that while human rights have been critical to enabling access, and as AIDS treatment has been firmly placed on the global policy agenda, there is evidence that enthusiasm for human rights in responses to AIDS is ebbing (Viljoen, and Precious 2007; see also Gruskin, Ferguson, Bogecho 2007; Pisani 2008). Above all, the book explores, through a case study, the complicated national and local forces and contexts that human rights and treatment programs must negotiate if they are to have greater relevance and sustained success. Rather than taking the easier option to simply drift away from human rights, as increasingly appears to be the case, it is argued that the messiness of social, political, and cultural relations must be engaged with. This engagement will be beneficial in strengthening both human rights approaches and AIDS treatment programs, including the likelihood of adherence to ARVs.

Against the Deafening Silence on AIDS Treatment

It is hard to comprehend that there was ever resistance and procrastination to the introduction of policy to expand access to AIDS treatment. Some actors in the policy process now reflect back on that period when support for expansion amongst donors was limited as an "absurd debate."(Piot, 2008). To this end, literally mountains—consisting of states, pharmaceutical companies, and above all, engrained political, cultural, and social attitudes—have had to be moved (A'desky 2004). One of the biggest obstacles was treatment skeptics, featuring donors, governments, and others who, only a short time ago, maintained that expansion or "rollout" of ARVs was politically and economically unworkable. In addition, many claimed that treatment was also culturally and socially inappropriate in low resource settings (See Jones 2004a). Put simply, expensive and sophisticated AIDS medication was deemed incompatible with "local standards of care."[2] Poverty, corruption, inequality, and cultural habits would all apparently lead to failure of treatment programs. These factors were therefore identified as likely to undermine a patient's ability to adhere to ARVs. Because of these concerns, from the beginning of global debate on expanding access to ARVs the issue of adherence has had a deep imprint upon AIDS treatment discourse and practice.

Human rights-based approaches to the epidemic, on the other hand, sought to combat this negativity and the exclusion it created by instead arguing that access to treatment was a fundamental human right. Struggles surrounding prevention, and then treatment and legal protection for people living with AIDS, have also given a tremendous galvanizing force to movements for health and human rights (Mann and Tarantola 1998).

In terms of struggles over medication, at its simplest, more than forty years ago, the International Covenant on Economic, Social and Cultural Rights had acknowledged the right to treatment as intrinsic to the human right to "the highest attainable level of physical and mental health," as were preventative aspects (see Chapter 2). In more recent years, supporters of the right to AIDS medication used this as a platform from which to argue that while medical knowledge and technology existed that could prolong lives, due to its high cost, it remained out of reach. Profiteering of pharmaceutical companies and the obstinance of states, so the argument went, should never be at the cost of the right to health and to life itself. Contrary to those opponents, a consensus began to emerge that most objections to extending treatment remained purely theoretical and therefore needed testing practically by actually *doing* treatment in so-called low resource settings. The urgency became ever more apparent as AIDS was identified as at the vanguard of a rapidly (re)emerging "ill-health curtain" drawn between the "First" and "Third" Worlds. This ill-health curtain is characterised by stark differences in health conditions, none starker, or more telling, than a dramatic AIDS-related decline in life expectancy and rising infant mortality a feature of many African countries (Heywood 2002:218; UNDP 2002).[3] Spurred on, then, by the devastatingly high burden of disease associated with the epidemic, the global momentum for extending treatment, cast in the image of human rights, became irresistible. It was the sustained pressure of treatment activists and their allies who laid bare the "deafening silence" of the more affluent parts of world in their indifference toward people living with AIDS on the other side of the "ill-health curtain" (Cameron 2000). This force culminated in worldwide protests against pharmaceutical companies and obstructive governments and leaders on both sides of the "curtain," and a series of global meetings, declarations of commitments, and international cooperation. The campaigning and global momentum contributed to a dramatic decline in drug prices that provided the catalyst for the treatment era to finally become reality in the so-called developing Global South.[4] Having settled, for now, some of the profound global policy battles to extend access, attention has increasingly focused upon in-country experiences of ARV "rollout."

Recent Phenomenon

A feature of the care and treatment of people living with AIDS in the West for over a decade, ARV medication is still a recent phenomenon for those living in the Global South. In 2004, upon gazing out my hotel window in the capital city of a Southern African country, metaphors for inequality were all too easily evident. It really was a long way down to the bustling street, adorned with purple blossoms cascading from the Jacaranda trees. A constant stream of cramped mini-kombi taxis en route to the sprawling townships beeped their horns to alert potential passengers. Wave after wave jostled with the handful of unfeasibly large four-wheel drive vehicles. Upon opening the daily newspaper, one of the stories was about a visiting group of overseas (Western) members of Parliament who reprimanded the country's citizens for not doing enough in their fight against corruption, stating that it could only be achieved if the residents worked hard to attain zero tolerance. How do you absorb such exhortations at the same time as you observe a Poverty Reduction Strategy meeting between the World Bank, European Union stakeholders, and members of the state elite that was taking place in the well-watered gardens of the hotel? Behind high and closed walls, secluded from the bustling streets and local markets, it was not hard to have doubts about the degree of popular accountability over deliberations that could ever possibly ensue at such an elitist transnational meeting. What would become of efforts to expand AIDS treatment in such a context?

These concerns weigh heavier still when one considers that in this country where 80 percent of residents are estimated to be living in poverty, the Secretary of State for Health declared in the newspaper that he was still only *considering* making ARVs free in the public health sector. The point is that these deliberations over macroeconomic policy and treatment were taking place at a time when AIDS activists told me about waiting lists for ARV treatment that seemed "never ending." A prolonged wait was deadly for those who were seriously ill and for those whose health deteriorated daily as they waited. Clinical criteria appeared to be the basis of eligibility for granting access to treatment. Moreover, such criteria, when following a "first-come, first-served" rationale, also appeared, at face value, to be intrinsically "fair" and nondiscriminatory. However, upon closer scrutiny, at the time of observation, the patient was required (until 2005) to pay a fee toward access to medication and associated tests. The urban, better connected, and more privileged were jumping these queues (and not because their medical conditions were necessarily any higher priority), with public debate on access apparently nonexistent. Class, geography, gender, bureaucracy, culture, and clinical criteria heavily circumscribed access here, as elsewhere, in the region.

So while global incantations of human rights appeared to make treatment an increasing reality, they were actually conditioned and constrained by various social, economic, political, clinical, and cultural facts on the ground. I considered how these issues, namely, human rights and the socioeconomic, political, cultural, and clinical context, play a role in shaping access to ARVs in regions such as Southern Africa. How the huge increase in resources and new determination of governments and donors to extend access to ARVs interacts with these kinds of dynamics, the unequal relations, and uneven state, civil society, and donor power appears to be an increasingly important issue for many countries in the Global South.

ARVs and Governance Networks

In the urgency to place people on treatment, efforts to expand access must also allow for some reflection. At times, this race appears to be a sprint toward the finishing line. To that end, holding governments to commitments to produce firm outputs—including numbers on treatment—has been admirable, refreshing, and necessary. More often than not, though, it has given the impression of an awkward three-legged race at a school sports event. The "legs" of states, market actors, and civil society organizations, seemingly tethered together by the rope of global norms and institutions, now comprise new transnational forms of decision making and partnerships. These networks are somewhat artificial assemblages, therefore, appearing to work toward common goals, yet with each actor seeking to protect their own agendas. The essence of these novel forms of AIDS governance is that they do not necessarily act in any predictable or consistently coordinated fashion. Above all, it is by no means easily apparent which of the actors are responsible for steering and pulling the participants along. Against the backdrop of huge increases in global AIDS funding, these new governance networks are now played out in very different country contexts. Such networks behold very different trajectories and implications for responses to HIV/AIDS, especially for putting, and keeping, people on treatment.

But the learning by doing has produced a very steep learning curve, one that has demonstrated not only that treatment is clearly "doable" but that it can also be highly successful (Heywood 2004). It also provides an opportunity, as suggested, to seek heightened reflection upon experiences of "scaling-up" treatment. At the same time as the implementation era for AIDS medication is increasingly a reality, a wide range of effects emerge from this era, thereby posing questions and challenges to both the scope and nature of treatment delivery and the relevance of a rights-based approach to it. This book is a contribution to creating such spaces of reflection upon, and critical understanding of, both AIDS treatment and human rights implementation. Both have been conjoined in struggles to access medication and their effects now require constructive scrutiny. One of the main issues addressed, therefore, is what locally-grounded struggles over access to medication can tell us more generally about the place of treatment in the epidemic and human rights in the twenty-first century. In such a politicized policy arena as this, the intention here is to seek to shed light upon the local (and national) contexts that treatment and rights must navigate in order that interventions become strengthened. There is still such a long way to go to ensure universal access. But just as a human rights-based approach was catalytic in creating policy to deliver ARVs to millions, now, however, the treatment era poses a number of challenges to responses to AIDS and human rights. Several paradoxes can be identified.

The Rise of Treatment and Human Rights Drift

What an irony, then, that before we can even say that a human rights approach was ever secured, it now appears to be losing favor, cast out as not working, or just plain difficult to achieve. Some of this disenchantment with rights in the context of disappointing responses to AIDS is due in part to the failure, as Gruskin et al (2007) suggest, in identifying easily comprehensible rights-based policy successes. The complicated amalgam of concepts and approaches encompassing a "rights-based approach" certainly does not tend to easily assist policy makers. Another source is simply that policy prescriptions constantly evolve: as another paradigm becomes less favored, another emerges. But, in addition, I would also suggest that wavering interest in human rights sees a drift away from "rights-based" responses not only to AIDS, but perhaps also more generally. It does not appear uncoincidental, for example, that as human rights and civil liberties are increasingly perceived globally as somehow soft on the "War on Terror" and threats posed by terrorism to national security, a rights-based focus is being depicted by international organizations, and states alike, as soft on the "War against AIDS." Rights—perceived by some as responsible for facilitating the spread of AIDS and/or enabling a permissive liberalism in conservative societies—are under threat (Viljoen and Precious 2007). The corollary being touted is the desire to return to what are perceived, wrongly, as more appropriate epidemiologically targeted and coercive health interventions (Pisani 2008). Before looking at some of the manifestations of what I term the "human rights drift," I turn first to a brief summary of the rise of treatment on the global scene.

The Place of Treatment Globally

One very visible indicator of the accelerated shift in global responses to the epidemic is the increase in flows of funding available to tackle HIV/AIDS. Once a seemingly insurmountable barrier, in 1996, global funds stood at approximately $300 million. By 2005, however, according to UNAIDS, there had been a massive twenty-eight-fold increase to around $8.3 billion.[5] Furthermore, spawned by campaigning, declarations, and commitments, there is now a distinctive AIDS architecture reflecting both human rights content and the novel (and not so novel) forms of governance networks mentioned. By 2005, again according to UNAIDS, bilateral assistance (funding given directly from one state to another) and multilateral funding (funding given indirectly via global institutions such as the World Bank and the Global Fund) represented 68.8 percent of total global funding for AIDS. This means that particular countries, notably the United States (which is by far the largest bilateral donor through its President's Emergency Plan for AIDS Relief, or, PEPFAR) and to a lesser extent, the United Kingdom, are particularly influential actors, especially for specific recipient countries.

But one of the most innovative departures from old patterns of disbursing aid has been the creation of the multilateral Global Fund. The fund has emerged as a very significant actor in the global distribution of AIDS funding, especially with its emphasis upon in-country partnership. Countries' own domestic sources of funding have also increased. Peter Piot estimates that approximately one-third of the total funding is now paid for by middle- and lower-income countries themselves. That some heavily aid-dependent and indebted countries pay such a large amount in proportion to their national income raises questions about whether this is morally acceptable (Piot 2008). Finally, there are other very significant private actors, such as charitable foundations, nongovernmental organizations, and businesses, including the pharmaceutical industry itself. The Bill and Melinda Gates Foundation, for example, is also a major private actor within these networks. There is now a quite bewildering array of partnership arrangements. Although there are notable efforts to coordinate these partnerships, such complicated constellations of funding, with different ideological, sectoral, and organizational requirements, inevitably qualify whether these "gifts" of aid are always benevolent under existing terms and conditions (Jones 2004b).[6] In other words, we should be considering that there is a geopolitics of treatment. Is there, for example, an inverse relationship between the vast increase in resources and loss of sovereignty and authority for recipient countries? And does the scale of intervention actually provoke particular governments to pursue policies in reaction to the perception or reality of erosion of control?

Within this constellation, between 2006–8, AIDS treatment and care was predicated by UNAIDS to require an estimated $12.3 billion. Treatment and care is second only to the largest funded component, prevention, at $29.8 billion. Within this predicted allocation needed for treatment and care, opportunistic infections reflect a significant component of the funding. As a recent addition, the amount for antiretrovirals themselves (that is, the drugs) now comprises more than half of all funding for treatment responses. When associated laboratory, logistical, and human resource costs and the rapid increase in the number of patients associated with ARVs are also factored in, then it is clear that treating AIDS has gone from being nonexistent to now comprising a huge and relatively recent component of total global AIDS expenditure. And this constellation, as suggested, takes on all shapes of AIDS governance trajectories and specific regional patterns. Southern Africa, for example, receives more than 55 percent of the treatment funding, and is especially characterized by donor dependency. Never before has the opportunity to extend life through ARVs been greater and never before has AIDS treatment occupied a more prominent global role.

Both in terms of the allocated finance and future requirements and also in terms of new directions in global responses to the epidemic, then, ARVs (and associated costs) have been exalted to a towering status. Some influential actors, such the chair of the Global HIV Prevention Working Group, describe the role of treatment as no less than "the best chance the world has had to build on a comprehensive response to the global epidemic. More widespread access to treatment is likely to bring millions of people into health care settings, providing new opportunities for health care workers to deliver and reinforce HIV prevention messages."[7] Underpinning such a response are associated claims made by the World Health Organization (WHO) that: "Universal access to antiretroviral therapy for everyone who requires it according to medical criteria opens up ways to accelerate prevention in communities in which more people will know their HIV status–and, critically, will *want* to know their status. As HIV/AIDS becomes a disease that can be both prevented and treated, attitudes will change, and denial, stigma and discrimination will rapidly be reduced. Rolling out effective HIV/AIDS treatment is the single activity that can most effectively energize and accelerate the uptake and impact of prevention." (WHO 2003b:6).

Following this line of logic, treatment will supposedly act as an incentive for people to come forward and test because they *want* to know their status. These are considerable claims, far over and above the moral and rights-based ones, for why people should be enabled access to treatment in the first place. These are claims demanding closer scrutiny, and ones that should be grounded within understanding of treatment services within specific local communities. But equally, alongside these good intentions, such as the emphasis upon "normalizing" HIV/AIDS, are more unintended consequences accompanying the treatment era.

Treatment and a Public Health Approach

In the global efforts to scale-up treatment, it is important to inquire as to the scope and nature of "access," and of its impact, particularly once treatment has been "accessed." For all the rights-based and participatory rhetoric of the WHO and UNAIDS treatment initiatives[8] and others, however, a public health model often, but not necessarily, ends up being reified.

In her excellent book, *City of Plagues*, Susan Craddock (Craddock 2000:3) makes the more general important point that it "is not to say that public health policies through the years have not been responsible for much that is beneficial, but it is to say that there is a sustained failure within medicine and public health to recognize the effect institutional practice has upon those suffering real or ascribed burdens of disease." Others go further in suggesting it is in spite of, and not because of, public health approaches that marginalized groups mobilize in the face of the epidemic (Stoller 1998). If the relationship between medical discourse, institutional practice, and the social and political roles of disease is not a new area of enquiry, then in terms of providing ARVs on a global scale, it is. There is a headlong rush to deliver ARV treatment. But, in doing so, it is pertinent to inquire whether the urgency and control of the process forsakes engagement with some of the less visible and complicated contexts that conditions patients' access. If so, what are some of the consequences, whether intended or unintended? How, as we will see, is public health entwined with these other paradoxes? And can these contexts be acknowledged and, as a consequence, communities placed on more progressive trajectories to tackle the epidemic?

Why Might Some People Not Want to Take ARVs?

"Eh! Some of the people are scared of treatment because . . . if you spoke to someone and say 'let us go and get some treatment' they will pretend as if they take it and then stop. They do not drink it" ("Thandi," female, Temba/Hammanskraal, South Africa).[9]

Apparently, outside many of the policy considerations, yet always a part of them, there is also a patient's own specific biographical context. Following the quotation above from a person living with AIDS in this book's South African case study area, one of the most obvious paradoxes is why, even when ARVs are available to some people, do they choose not to take them? How do we explain such decisions governing taking treatment? Are these decisions shaped at the level of the individual or are they also part of a web of social relations that span the family, community, and institutions, and even nation-building? How does this broader context shape the way people get treatment? And how does it influence the manner in which the treatment is taken, perhaps, as in the quotation above, in pretending to take it? While drawing on several experiences across a range of countries, this book is ultimately aimed at locating such treatment decision making within the dynamics of a specific local community. Exploring the mosaic of socioeconomic, cultural, political, and institutional relations in the South African community of Hammanskraal-Temba serves to place AIDS treatment in its appropriate context.

Treatment Displacing Prevention and Rights

There are other paradoxes that can now be associated with the treatment era. In order to fulfill access to treatment as a human right, for example, certain civil and political rights—particularly having to do with testing—are eroding (AIDS and Rights Alliance for Southern Africa 2006). Doctors remain frustrated that, in many countries, patients only come forward for testing and treatment when they are already so ill that it decreases the chances of a successful outcome. Many doctors therefore call for more proactive routine testing being offered by providers. While apparently sounding reasonable, and most would agree that uptake of testing is important, debate rages about the appropriate mode of testing to do so. The pros and cons of routine testing are discussed, with disagreement about whether patients need to "opt in" or "opt out" of the test and how such forms of testing might be open to abuse. In particular there are signs of increasing pressure to dispense with consent and counseling, which threatens to undermine a patient's coping ability.[10]

The medical rationale driving routine (and, from some quarters, mandatory) testing is also that such approaches are necessary in order to dislodge the stubborn social components associated with AIDS, namely, fear and stigma, which inhibits people from testing and seeking treatment. It is pertinent to reiterate Craddock's warning of the "effect institutional practice has upon those suffering real or ascribed burdens of disease." Caution is expressed about the role of treatment, therefore, in that it may serve to deemphasize prevention efforts and in fact leave these stubborn and resilient social attitudes untouched (Sozi in Jones 2007).[11] Peter Piot, Director of UNAIDS until 2009, while praising the success of placing more than 3 million on treatment in a relatively short time period, nonetheless laments that for every two people put on treatment, another five become infected. The pace of treatment is being outstripped by new infections in what some term a failure of prevention (Piot 2008). Treatment may not change the community and social contexts like the relations between men and woman, attitudes toward sex, and so on, that, according to Campbell (2003), led to the development of the epidemic in the first place. In a nutshell, in the "treatment era" can a medicine therefore really succeed in dislodging the deeply entrenched stigmatizing attitudes that surround sexuality, race, class, and gender associated with AIDS? Far from dislodging these social drivers of the epidemic, some even suggest that a renewed medicalization of AIDS through treatment is serving to reinforce them or at least demoting preventative efforts.[12] Others also point to the role of ARVs in changing sexual behavior, hence rebounding upon prevention efforts.

In the treatment era, some governments now find it more convenient to skirt around controversial issues having to do with, for example, sexuality, sex workers, and intravenous drug-taking because they can point to treatment programs as their principal policy commitment. In Zambia, for example, Catherine Sozi, the UNAIDS country representative describes this as follows: "It [treatment] was about getting the drugs and technical issues to get them, whereas prevention raises moral issues and is trickier . . . The rate of disclosure [in Zambia] is not high. There is political commitment, yes, but not private commitment. The dialogue on the private level is missing. Policies may be in place but people don't buy in privately."[13]

Treatment campaigns, such as WHO's "3 by 5" initiative, may unwittingly contribute to reimposing a dominant biomedical model upon responses to the epidemic. Concrete evidence for such emerges from an in-depth ethnological account of Brazil's response. In this, Biehl (2007:135) notes the impact of what he calls the pharmaceuticalization of public health. This, he suggests, has led to the emphasis on access to ARVs displacing state-provided prevention and clinical care. Another key paradox, therefore, is that as rights are being claimed and new subjectivities are being created by AIDS patients, the strong public institutions needed in the care of the most vulnerable are disappearing at all levels of government in Brazilian health and social care. With significance for aid-dependent countries, even in this non-aid-dependent country, in a neo-liberal era, it is still no coincidence that civil society, state and private sector partnerships have become the leading *modus operandi* to deliver treatment. In a trade-off, civil society may have gained influence within state policymaking but local care groups now occupy the gaps left in state provision. In encountering resource limitations, these organizations have become "a venue for incipient AIDS public health triage system." As a result, the poorest and most socially disadvantaged are being excluded from any follow-up.

The net impact is that treatment and associated scaling-up of testing services has the consequence, in many places, of eroding public voice and accountability surrounding the epidemic. This is because delivery is now being done to passive, privatized patients, with these stubborn and sensitive issues sidelined with implications also for prevention (Imrie, Elford, Kippax, and Hart 2007). Whereas access for the working and middle classes is enabled, new inequalities arise because the vulnerable are not supported. In addition to the social politics associated with AIDS, public health approaches to treatment should therefore also have cognizance of the ways they may lend themselves to shaping influential political and discursive interpretations of the epidemic. And, in all of these treatment interventions, can we, as Campbell concurs, say with any certainty that communities have actually been strengthened in dealing with the epidemic?

Other effects of the "treatment era" can be identified. For example, some observers highlight how treatment has lent itself to a drive to "normalize" HIV/AIDS, which is to seek to transform it into a manageable chronic illness, shorn of its stigmatizing connotation of death. While clearly laudable, such a desire is also replete with ambiguity. "Normalization" may be at the vanguard of a new form of (self-) disciplining of and (self-) control by people living with AIDS: "On the one hand, treatment addresses the reality of biological illness, the fear of dying and the stigma associated with a lethal disease. But at the same time, the transformation of AIDS into a manageable chronic illness can be part of a process whereby PWAs [people with AIDS] are tacitly instructed that they have no right to complain about their predicament: treatment is available, as are a vast array of additional health resources earmarked for HIV-sufferers." (Robins 2005:22).

Emphasis, for example, is placed upon patients who do not comply or adhere to medication, labeling them as irresponsible and to blame for their own predicament. In this way, as Farmer notes, noncompliance, or likelihood of noncompliance, becomes a tool to deny access, repackaged as "a rational public health strategy." While few would deny the importance of adherence, as will be shown in Chapter 2, it is, after all, those "who are least likely to comply who are those least likely to comply." In other words, whether Brazil or South Africa, those finding it most difficult to comply are likely to encounter more barriers than most. And rather than dealing with this, it may instead become a slippery slope between noncompliance and its use in justifying,[14] or indirectly limiting, access to medication.

Another outcome of this new form of patient governance has been witnessed in countries having longer and well-established ARV access, with a depoliticizing effect that treatment is having upon political and social activism.[15] Biehl describes the transition to "patient-citizenship" amongst the most marginalized people in Brazil's cities. He regards it as something of a trade-off between "disciplining" patients so they adhere, hence improving their chances of survival, but with social and political consequences: "This practice of citizenship via patienthood (or at least a claim to it) would transform in the subsequent years—at an impressive speed—into a very focused and sophisticated practice of care for one's pharmaceutical well-being. These individuals and their AIDS community would become less confrontational with political forces, less inclined to street life, and more integrated with the life-guaranteeing mechanisms and technologies associated with AIDS policy, local and national" (Biehl 2007:302–3).

These reflections suggest that normalization has impacted upon AIDS activism. Movements have been defused, whether by a politics of survival or more blatant co-option. For other observers, like de Waal, who now seek explanations for why AIDS has not precipitated the political crisis that he and others predicated for Africa, the role of activism features prominently. De Waal (2006) suggests that the important global constellations that I mentioned earlier and the adoption of a rights-based agenda have largely accommodated the aims and objectives of activists. One outcome is that activist approaches are inherently about reform rather than any revolution in social or political relations. That is, AIDS activism is not about seeking to overthrow poorly performing governments (even in South Africa). Instead, a reformist agenda has been promoted, and one that might even provide succor to regimes rather than tackling the root causes and politics that continue to drive the epidemic.

State Power and AIDS

With this in mind, another important dimension conditioning the political impact of AIDS concerns, as mentioned, is the huge amount of AIDS-oriented development resources flowing into regions, especially Southern Africa, in the last ten years. And, related to this, the type of partnerships that states and civil societies encourage, or are encouraged to form by donors, is significant. These partnership arrangements are used to gain leverage over decision making, sometimes to confront pharmaceutical companies and vested interests in order to lower prices, but more usually to access the development funds and, in association, enable political survival. The political impact of this funding is still to be fully charted. But one recent attempt shows that some governments and recipient NGOs have levered this funding for their own political ends (de Waal 2006). Economic benefits and political capital accrued due to the epidemic have contributed to regime survival.

For those with some insight into development aid and its uses and abuses, this will not come as any surprise. But it nonetheless requires scrutinizing how it has been used, filtered, and manipulated by different agendas in the context of AIDS. Some African leaders, for example, notably President Museveni in Uganda, have been able to generate international acclaim for proactive preventative responses to, and apparent reduction in, prevalence. Although disputed, and with the reasons for decrease in prevalence poorly understood, it has heightened the international standing of Museveni. Again, innovative new multisector networks of governance have enabled an apparently successful response to HIV/AIDS in Uganda (Jones and Koffeld 2008). But this same network also served to act as a diversion from some political difficulties and unevenness of responses to AIDS in that country. Political commitment, as such, can be fragile and reversible. State responses and their place in AIDS governance networks therefore tell us much about the political, bureaucratic–and often donor dependent–characteristics of the state in question (Patterson 2006). Indeed, there is growing awareness of the political dynamics of the epidemic and the need to explain state responses.

These responses, as mentioned, also reveal a keen awareness of some state leaders and bureaucracies of the need to build new inclusive forms of cross-sectoral networks premised upon civil society and state partnerships. In other parts of the world, in Brazil for example, from early in the epidemic, common ground was built between activists and government. These partnership approaches came to characterize policy responses based upon mutual progressive commitment (Biehl 2007:61). State activism and grassroots and NGO organizations therefore forged efficient partnerships. Whilst this proved to be phenomenally successful in extending access to medication, Biehl demonstrates how the social and economic circumstances of the poorest and most vulnerable in Brazil's cities still endure unacceptably high levels of mortality. In relation, he therefore suggests that treatment outcomes are unequal and can only be properly understood in the context of three predominant forces mediating ARVs.

First, the changing organization of states has had consequences for the poorest in Brazil. Neoliberal state reform claws back resources for health care and considers prevention to be a private rather than public matter. The poorest, Biehl observes, has in effect been abandoned.

Second, pharmaceutical companies and the market in fact undergo more, and not less, institutionalization. As if to capture this development, mention is made of how pharmaceutical companies dramatically impact government spending, with over two-thirds of Brazil's ARV budget going to these companies. There is also the growing influence of drug companies through "Pharma philanthropy," which has embedded itself more deeply within states and societies, influencing drug regimens, for example.

Third, patient-driven political demands, as suggested, are transformed into biological-based rights concerned with a micropolitics of survival. Biomedical intervention reflects a medicalization of marginalization. If this is taking place within Brazil, so influential in terms of the global efforts to extend access, we should surely be scrutinizing the broader impact of global funding elsewhere in the world. Crudely put, as AIDS organizations and activists sit with the state in collaboration, they begin to justify, in Brazil, both state polices and, more alarmingly, themselves.[16]

As suggested earlier, this should not come as a surprise because the history of development interventions, generally, has tended toward a litany of delivery being modernizing, technical, top-down, and depoliticizing in their effect (Ferguson 1992). Furthermore, in the contemporary era, such interventions are more likely to be about state-centered, elite institutional reforms devoid of local substantive democratization.[17] Rather than being overly obsessed with the formal attributes of democracy–such as voting and strong institutions—a more substantial definition "emphasises the introduction of democratic principles, institutions and citizenship rights" (Harriss et al 2004:6). The de Waal discourse on *AIDS and Power*, as relevant as it is, actually underscores a broader, more general need for critical engagement between the AIDS "sector" and progressive development more generally. It is not merely to cite and critique the reformist agenda of "rights"–by which de Waal seems to imply that a more revolutionary rupture is the solution to Africa's problems—but to insist upon democratization. Such a vision of deeper democracy should foreground human rights and institutions that have real meaning for people, and critically, can be used by them to strengthen democratic accountability. How the provision of

AIDS funding and treatment now plays out in the context of struggles over democratization is therefore of fundamental importance in understanding state responses to the epidemic.

In 2002, for example, the Botswana government took the incredibly visionary medical step forward to introduce the first ever public sector AIDS treatment program in Africa. In doing so, it is undeniable that the Botswana government forever broke the mold of the low expectations concerning treatment in Africa. The government promotes itself as having the best treatment program in Africa. But even as it does so, concerns have been raised by civil society about the extent to which the medicalization of the response to AIDS in Botswana has served to reinforce a kind of hardening in political and policymaking "space" between the state and civil society. In effect, the treatment program may be negatively changing such relationships: "The ARV era has generated arrogance from government. It closes room for learning more. They want to think they are the best" (Executive Secretary, Botswana Network of AIDS Service Organizations, BONASO).[18] The quotation captures well the apparent collusion between treatment (and related testing and other services) interventions and political effects and uses of such programs.

When set against the earlier backdrop of the pre-ARV era in low resource settings, whereby doctors could write only death certificates, it might appear trite to raise such issues. And in many countries, like South Africa, as we will see, civil society and state partnerships such as those existing in Brazil, could only be dreamt about. After all, none of this was ever an argument against treatment becoming a humanitarian intervention—a lived reality, offering life, hope, and dignity for millions of people living with AIDS—than would otherwise be the case in its absence. And whilst policy responses may in some cases be co-opted for specific agendas treatment has also served as a site of social and political struggle that injected considerable global momentum into rights-based advocacy, and social and community mobilization directed toward the ends of social justice and measurable outcomes of governments.

Even in terms of warnings of the reinscription of a dominant biomedical model upon tackling the epidemic, there are interesting spaces for contestation from within. A range of more progressive alternatives exists. Paul Farmer, for example, drawing on his long experience of working in Haiti with *Partners in Health*, questions whether doctors are in fact the most efficient distributors of ARVs. Instead, Farmer suggests a need to promote more creative alternatives, such as well-trained community health workers, whom he claims are more appropriate for addressing important social issues as much as medical ones (Justice Africa 2007). And other community-based initiatives—such as the exemplary one of the *Treatment Action Campaign* (TAC) in South Africa—are directed toward community-based activism and treatment literacy as important tools to democratize scientific knowledge. Communities exposed to such organizing can cope better with the epidemic (TAC 2007).There has been heightened awareness of the need and benefits in creating "new social subjects" and "responsibilized" citizens who can turn the negative attributes of AIDS into more constructive meanings and belonging. Most impressively, people living with AIDS are fashioning new AIDS identities, drawing upon the increasing availability of ARVs, AIDS activism, solidarity, and the quasi-religious revelation found in reversing near-death experiences (Robins 2004).

Nonetheless, difficult questions still remain about what the impacts of such interventions are having, even within these more progressive spaces. Critical questions directed at responses to the epidemic, and specifically, scaling up of treatment and testing, remain inescapably valid. This validity in turn vexes us to conceptualize a response to the following questions: what is a successful treatment program and what does or should it look like?

How to Measure Success?

Certainly, some may suggest that success lies in the hard numbers on treatment, ideally in genuinely universal access. But many others would surely point to scrutinizing its quality. But what then constitutes quality? The MASA (meaning "new dawn") treatment program in Botswana presents what appear to be indicators of an incredibly successful outcome: eight out of ten patients who walk through the clinic doors survive and benefit from ARV treatment; one out of ten is lost to mortality; and another one in ten is lost to "follow-up" (i.e., they fall out of the public treatment system) (Jones 2007). In terms of a very high adherence—higher than people living with AIDS in the West—and successful medical outcomes, from a medical point of view, it perhaps cannot get too much better. This appears to be the epitome of a successful program. But while the next section qualifies its success, even if medical efficacy is the paramount goal and if we accept that a person's *attitude* toward treatment impacts upon its acceptance and use (Schrimshaw, Siegel, and Lekas 2005), then a full spectrum of social, political, economic, and cultural factors must be taken into consideration to understand such outcomes.

The former head of MASA, for example, could not explain what had happened to those 10 percent of patients who had been lost to "follow-up." Nor could she say what has happened to stigma *outside* of the clinic doors. And, in claiming that stigma inside the clinics had dissipated, she then informed me about a "caring for carers" program, working with health care workers to counsel, test, and treat them. This was in response to "many" cases of nurses and doctors falling ill, collapsing even, in the work place before finally having to confront their status and the nature of their illness. In other words, the claim made by some that stigma ends at the ARV clinic door appears inaccurate. Those supposedly closest to information and treatment, namely, health care workers, shun acceptance. And their denial apparently underscores the resilience of stigma associated with HIV/AIDS. One also needs to go beyond the eight out of ten figures, as impressive as this is, to also ask qualitative questions about how, and with what impact, the patient discovered their status, and how it is to live on treatment in their community. Again, as BONASO put it: "With '3 X 5' we all got carried away with treatment, with building laboratories, and so on, and we forgot about prevention. So we should not leave rights behind or the needs of the client."[19] This comment neatly sums up some of the tensions involved in implementing the right to treatment. On the one hand, there is a drive toward building infrastructure and getting patients to drugs and drugs to patients. But this should not be at the sake of impinging on other related rights and needs of the client in the context of access to health care and accountability over decision making, on the other hand. Indeed, there is a lack of recourse to rights-based provisions in Botswana, with very limited specific legal protection for people living with AIDS and other vulnerable groups.

Furthermore, even treatment coverage figures (for example, percentage of people living with AIDS who could benefit from ARVs and who actually have access to them) are contested. Some civil society organizations in Botswana dispute the WHO figure of 85 percent coverage, and even the government's own figure of 75 percent. Some instead suggest the figure is around 40 percent. Even well placed actors in the treatment program place coverage at more likely around 67 percent.[20] So the question of access still remains paramount not only for those on treatment but also the 33 percent *not* accessing it, many of whom might also face additional hurdles as "hard to reach" groups. The patient, and potential patient, is, after all, embedded in a web of complex social relations governing access and use of treatment.

In a similar vein, I have deliberately chosen to be up-front about adherence figures in the case study subject area of the book. This is in order to challenge what it is we think treatment programs should be doing, to divert focus from adherence levels *per se*. I did not want to write a case study of important contextual issues only for it to culminate in rendering adherence as the key measure of success and failure. For while few would contest the public health claim and common objective that it is a priority that patients are kept alive, the point should also be how treatment interplays with the social politics of the epidemic. In other words, what can treatment do and not do? Rather than asking about what all the dynamics to come in the chapters imply for adherence levels, I prefer to say something about them here. These were also hard to ascertain due to lack of data at the local clinic in the case study area. Dr. Mathibedi, head of *Wellness* ARV clinic, suggested that approximately 70 percent of patients were "benefiting" from ARVs, whilst 30 percent were not.[21] This does not, of course, tell us anything about what proportion of patients are retained (that is, patients known to be alive and receiving ARVs at the end of a follow-up period), over what kind of time span, or how many are lost to attrition (those who discontinue use of ARVs). In other words, a 70 percent estimate of benefit—and hence adherence—does not give any indication of whether the patient cohort is losing patients, for whatever reasons, although this can be inferred. Indeed, in a study of a range of treatment programs across Africa to date, on average, the programs achieved 60 percent patient retention after two years. Within more than half of the programs, the main factor in the majority of all incidents of attrition was given as "lost to follow-up" (a specified time after which patients are late for a scheduled consultation or pick-up for medication). Patient tracking is therefore a key consideration to find out more about attrition.[22] But based on other evidence from South African treatment sites, a 70 percent retention level would not necessarily appear to be inaccurate for the *Wellness* ARV clinic.

Although this figure was not broken down into the reasons for why treatment was not proving beneficial for the 30 per cent in question, the clinic indicated that the biggest factor in the majority of cases was adherence problems. Dr. Mathibedi predicted that these figures were likely to worsen, rather than improve, as a new generation of treatment users emerged. A downward pressure upon adherence rates was explained in terms of a generational shift in patients. Many newer patients increasingly access treatment at a stage before they encounter the near-death experiences that the first generation of patients has been dealing with. The inference was that unlike more recent patients, those near death experiences had produced a more zealous and near religious conversion to adherence—a second chance at life and hence was a major contributory factor in high levels of adherence. These are important issues, not least because the focus upon successful medical outcomes belies a central paradox of the treatment era: ARV treatment is an increasing reality for those who could benefit from it. But are those individual and community needs, rights-based approaches to tackle social stigma; political will and social mobilization, which drove the breakthroughs in treatment in the first place, being overridden by biomedical, technical and apolitical "solutions" to the epidemic?

Treatment's Grey Areas

In South Africa, studies are now beginning to explore the broader context in which to flesh out the grey areas of the "treatment era." They mainly focus upon the significant challenge, for example, of patient retention and how this determines successful treatment outcomes for the patient. Concerning whether retention is successful, one important study correlates levels of success with codetermining factors, such as quality of social support, substance and alcohol abuse, level of income, and stigma (Booysen, Anderson and Meyer 2006). Treatment activists and other actors hoped that the advent of ARVs would mean that the disease would no longer be associated with death (Heywood n.d., 23–25). But whether this has been the case is assessed in Chapter 5. And to illustrate the broader context of poverty and hardship in influencing decision making regarding treatment, Leclerc-Madlala (2006) looks specifically at the role of disability grants. Simply put, while the state decrees discontinuation of the grant as a patient's health improves, and also following an annual review by the Department of Social Development, this is identified as a disincentive to continuing treatment. The material factors impacting treatment behavior are therefore raised as a matter of urgency (Chapter 7). And even after treatment has been introduced free of charge into the public sector, this has not necessarily made expensive alternative medicines any less attractive to people living with AIDS (Chapter 6).

Another study found lack of enthusiasm for ARVs in some communities as well as fierce competition to ARVs from "alternative" products (Chopra et al 2006). Whilst the study here deliberately falls short of showing detailed (patient cohort-type) impact upon adherence, it does suggest that, over and above structural factors, complex personal, political, and community sociocultural attitudes are integral to a user, or potential user's, perception of ARVs. A rapidly developing literature is therefore taking stock of different readings of the epidemic itself, over and beyond the more obvious denialist views of prominent leaders in South Africa. Anthropologists and other social scientists have been at the forefront, investigating the role of cultural understandings of health and illness. Alternative explanations of death and illness in a context of AIDS surface social and cultural perceptions of cause rather than biological or physical ones (Posel, Kahn, and Walker 2007). Witchcraft is one amongst many beliefs associated with traditional beliefs but which are mediated in a context of rapid social change. Serious attention requires that analysis be freed from any understanding that attempts to capture culture as innate, or timeless. Witchcraft, for example, shouldnot be read as "an index of primitive ignorance and superstition" but instead rather as "an idiom through which other realities are expressed, realities such as social stress and strain, unemployment, capitalist globalization, the collective fantasizing of popular culture, and so on . . . [it] is not really about witches but is simply finding an idiom for expressing meaning of [in the case study discussed in Ashforth's book] his misfortune as an unemployed black man missing the gravy train in the new South Africa"(Ashforth 2000:245).

Understanding such perceptions is increasingly deemed integral to creating more successful policy interventions, public health and otherwise. In recognizing contested understandings of the nature and cause(s) of HIV/AIDS-related illness and death, logically, then, one would assume there must also be very different readings of "treatment."

Some of these dynamics are captured in Liz McGregor's powerful book, *Khabzela: Life and times of a great South African*, the poignant story of YFM ("Youth FM" radio) disc jockey, Fani Khabzela, and his untimely death from AIDS. In early 2003, Khabzela, according to the account pieced together by McGregor, was showing signs of illness. He revealed his status to listeners—one of the few public celebrities to do so—and was signed off on sick leave in April of that year. The expectation and hope of his employers was that he would commence ARVs and return to work within weeks. In contrast to the majority of people living with AIDS who were denied access to ARVs in the public health system at that time, ARVs were part of a generous medical care package financed by his employers. What took place instead, in January 2004, less than a year later, was Khabzela's spiraling descent into illness, which culminated in his death in the Johannesburg General Hospital. So here was someone who had considerable support—both financial and, given his disclosure, even emotional—but who chose to shun use of ARVs:

> He [Khabzela] did n't want to hear anything about anti-retrovirals. He did n't want to hear the words "anti-retrovirals". Sis Angie [a carer and AIDS counsellor] was saying to him "Look drink the herbs but also drink the anti-retrovirals because anti-retrovirals are made specifically to deal with the virus within you, to fight the virus. The herbs are good to boost your immune system". He took [the anti-retrovirals] for a week. He said he was getting worse. It was in his mind that they are going to kill him. So they could n't do much in his body because he did n't believe in them. After a week, he said: "No more anti-retrovirals. Say anti-retrovirals and I'm going to scream". He never took them again. They were just lying there in the house.[23]

Khabzela rejected ARVs, and McGregor attempts to identify some of the complex factors driving this person away from them and instead toward "alternative treatments." What followed was an odyssey of alternative treatments, such as consultations with *sangomas*, spiritualism, an herbal remedy put into pill form by someone medically unqualified to do so, and a nurse, apparently sent by the Minister of Health to administer a concoction of lemon juice and olive oil to be used with pills (*Africa's Solution*), with extracts from the African potato. A circus appeared around Khabzela. And while we can condemn the blatant opportunism of some of those wanting to make a name for themselves on the back of this individual's suffering, what is less contestable is that Khabzela had an ambivalence, at best, to ARVs, and at worst, an outright mistrust.

How people use, misuse, or in Khabzela's case, may choose not to use ARVs in preference instead for alternative treatment—some traditional, some not, and some spiritual—surely must challenge some of the grandiose claims made on behalf of treatment and the individual-rational model associated with it. The task placed before us, no less, is therefore that urged by Leclerc-Madlala: "While the need for a more contextually-sensitive model of behaviour change as an alternative to traditional individual decision-making model has been recognised in the context of HIV prevention in South Africa . . . there remains a need for such models in the era of AIDS treatment" (Leclerc-Madlala 2006).

This book seeks to fill in some of this broader context comprising treatment behavior. It does so by documenting and analyzing such "downstream" factors in order to unpack some of the subtleties and nuances to ARV rollout from the point of view of people living with AIDS themselves. And, moreover, it places access to ARVs in relation to a specific nation-building, service-delivery, and community setting. Indeed, the interface between patients and locally embedded institutions is a vital, yet hitherto ignored, arena governing access to treatment and services more generally (Chapter 4). Locally grounded evidence is developing but is still scarce. And because these problems are inherently complex and interrelated "joined-up problems," they require a multidisciplinary lens through which to understand them and to identify "joined-up" solutions. This book is a modest attempt to contribute to these endeavors. It is intended to elaborate on the meaning of "access" to treatment in order to produce a more rounded picture of the dilemmas, anxieties, community, and institutional and contextual pressures—the gray areas—that people-living-with-AIDS encounter. A key recurring theme is the linkage between, on the one hand, an individual's decision-making process, predisposition to human rights, and the broader community and institutional context governing access to treatment on the other, both before *and* after treatment is accessed.

Synopsis of Chapters

In addition to the introduction and conclusion, the book is centered upon seven chapters. Chapter 1 provides an overview of the *struggle for treatment* in South Africa, whose defining characteristic has been one of heavy contestation. Not least, key figures in government—including the president and minister of health—have sought to interpret and locate the AIDS epidemic in the context of an Africanist nation-building project premised upon a broader vision of African Renaissance. Denialist explanations of the epidemic have been apparent and conventional scientific knowledge—particularly concerning the progression from HIV to AIDS—has been refuted. Of particular interest for what follows is how ARV medication became entwined with this elite- and some grassroots-driven project. ARVs have been treated with deep suspicion and outright hostility, with a state bias, until very recently, toward promotion of traditional and alternative medications. This contested backdrop provides an important context for understanding prevailing social attitudes toward ARVs and cultural beliefs—such as those expressed by ANC leader Jacob Zuma in this chapter and explored in more detail in other chapters. But Chapter 1 also locates AIDS treatment and the mounting disquiet over the position government preferred to take on it within the deep well of frustration surrounding service delivery more generally in South Africa. Countrywide protests over service delivery are indicative of deep-seated concerns over the direction of the country's development path and especially the erosion of citizen leverage over services, including access to ARVs.

Chapter 2 seeks to unpack *the meaning of "access"* to ARVs and human rights. It does so by placing access to essential medication within a useful rights-based framework, which has been pivotal to affirming the right to medication. But human rights as concept and practice are far from unambiguous, as also discussed. The chapter breaks down access in terms of the "availability" of medication and then elaborates on its "accessibility" in terms of financial, geographic, social, cultural, information, and institutional considerations. Influential global treatment programs, such as the WHO "3 by 5" campaign, have provided important momentum in terms of both conceptual and operational dimensions involved in extending access to ARVs. And the chapter therefore also suggests that ethical dimensions are important in terms of distributive justice of scarce resources. A critical entry point, whether implicitly or explicitly stated, is treatment guidelines. These, it is argued, should be carefully scrutinized so that they provide inclusion rather than exclusion of patients. A fundamental issue in access concerns the prevailing public health emphasis upon adherence or likelihood of adherence as the key determinant in initiating someone into treatment. This is inherently about medical efficacy rather than other ethical principles discussed. The chapter therefore looks in detail at South Africa's guidelines in order to illustrate some of these trade-offs and dilemmas.

Chapter 3 introduces the specific context in which to explore how these broader dynamics and issues are played out, namely through the case study area of *Hammanskraal-Temba*. The residue of apartheid planning and (racial, economic, geographic, and ethic) exclusion continues to condition the area. Not least, in the postapartheid era, service delivery is of critical concern for residents, and for community and state relations. The chapter therefore briefly looks at the historical development of Hammanskraal-Temba in order to identify key characteristics of the area. Since 1994, the era of liberation appears to increasingly give way to a politics of patronage at the local level, and one that exacerbates uneven efforts to extend services and opportunities to disadvantaged communities. The largest political support locally is undoubtedly for the ruling ANC. However, the coalition of groups centred upon the ANC which comprise formal political decision-making, it is argued, has contradictory implications for the quality of local democracy. This area has also witnessed rioting over service delivery. Such protests are symptomatic of residents' perception that they are not receiving the services they should, they are excluded from decision-making and that there is a lack of adequate accountability over decision-makers.

Chapter 4 brings these issues to bear upon provision of ARV medication in the local area. How *the organizational culture of the local hospital*—a place, it is argued, where authoritarianism and exclusion were vested under previous and current regimes—effects treatment rollout is the paramount concern. The chapter explores why some people living with AIDS perceive seeking treatment at this hospital as a "gamble." The catalog of violations of patient rights goes some way in explaining such a perception. And a specific focus is therefore how institutional structures serve to condition access to ARVs. Attempts are made to identify the source of the maltreatment of people living with AIDS, whether the difficult working conditions of health care workers, local social and cultural characteristics, or all of these and failure to have any redress through affirming rights. One damaging outcome is that the clinic appears to be prevented from working more closely with the community and sectoral collaboration is prevented by hospital management. Reciprocally, the community appears to detach itself from the hospital.

Chapter 5 assesses the prevailing views of ARVs in this community to explore whether the medication is deemed *socially acceptable*. The contested nature of ARVs rears itself in the context of the continuing stigma attached to AIDS. Contrary to expectations that ARVs would erode the stigma, it appears to be transferred onto the medication itself. ARVs have an image problem. Both this and the stigmatizing attitudes serve to constrain the ability of people living with AIDS to take the medication, with many often taking it in secret. But it also illustrates that deep-seated social attitudes and private and individual denial about the epidemic remains largely intact in this community. The chapter also looks at the role of information in influencing access. It should mitigate these fears but unfortunately appears to exacerbate the image problems of ARVs. The responsibility of leaders to provide unambiguous and accurate information is apparent and is urgently needed in this community.

Chapter 6 looks at the other key aspect in acceptability of ARVs, that is, *cultural acceptability*. The chapter shows how ARVs, in effect, must compete with a range of traditional and alternative medications. The relationship between elite-driven promotion of such alternatives and locally rooted beliefs is not always unidirectional. Although legitimate and popular leaders are clearly very influential in contributing to prevailing attitudes, the chapter suggests that the issue of cultural acceptability goes far beyond what elites may say or not say. These practices are very widespread, intergenerational, and trusted. However, it is also shown how this community reflects a large degree of confusion over such alternatives to ARVs. Some practices place vulnerable groups, such as children, at particularly high levels of risk. Many patients also choose to mix both types of medications. In particular, many of these alternatives are now driven by business motives that exploit vulnerable people living with AIDS. Nonetheless, for all the dilemmas, the rationale for why people take traditional and alternative medication is clear and the benefits are explored in the remainder of the chapter.

Chapter 7 situates treatment decisions within the context of both socioeconomic issues that present barriers to access and the role of clinical criteria currently being operationalized by the local clinic. The chapter looks at who is getting, but also finding it difficult to get, treatment. People living with AIDS themselves are asked whether the procedure to get treatment is easy or otherwise. These findings are then correlated to socioeconomic barriers such as physical distance, transport costs, and other associated barriers to do with food, water, and social grants. The main treatment guideline criteria examined is the one concerning disclosure. This resonates with Chapter 2 and the significance given to placing emphasis upon adherence. How disclosure criteria are applied in the clinic setting is looked at. One difficult issue is whether those people living with AIDS who have the least support are being filtered out of the procedure to access treatment.

The concluding chapter returns to the question of how both rights and ARV treatment programs should be better connected to communities and used to tackle broader forces driving the epidemic itself. How treatment can be made the platform for a genuine rights-based approach to the epidemic holds out great possibilities but also immense challenges. By necessity, such an approach must confront different expressions of power—whether institutional, political, cultural, social, or economic—that has always accompanied the epidemic. Are human rights up to this challenge?

CHAPTER 1

The Struggle to Access Treatment and Other Services in South Africa

In 2003, the South African government made a historic policy announcement to provide antiretroviral treatment (ARVs) in the public sector. With the subsequent Comprehensive Plan for HIV and AIDS Care, Management and Treatment, South Africa had apparently arrived in the treatment era. Years of discord between the state and civil society gave way to a national treatment plan and renewed hope for people living with AIDS, albeit metered by civil society's caution. After all, there is compelling evidence to suggest that the government's hand has been forced on AIDS policy. Outright denial and lingering skepticism have been long-standing features of the government's response to the epidemic (Nattrass 2004; Heywood 2005; Mbali 2004; Jones 2005a). In assessing the tortured path of AIDS policy in South Africa, Nattrass provides a fair indictment that it is "a sorry tale of missed opportunities, inadequate analysis, bureaucratic failure and political mismanagement" (Nattrass 2004:40).

So although the government has recently started to boast about its ARV programme as being the biggest (and best) in the world, perhaps one of the most telling indicators of the failures is the "treatment gap" in South Africa. The treatment plan subsequently adopted in November 2003 does build the foundation for the most extensive ARV program in the world, with a target of more than 1 million people on treatment by 2007–8. Implementation of the plan, however, has been criticized due to the slow rollout of treatment. The initial target to have 53,000 people on treatment by March 31, 2004, was postponed to the following year. By the beginning of April 2005, there were still only about 33,000 people who had been put on treatment.[1] Despite good policies and "gold standard" human rights-based legislation addressing HIV/AIDS, the implementation of the plan does not seem to be sufficiently prioritized. More recently, however, access has gained momentum. But still, in the first half of 2007, this "treatment gap"—the difference between numbers on ARVs in the public sector (257,108) and those that should be on ARVs according to the Department of Health's Operational Plan (716,771)—is estimated at 459,663, or 64 percent of those in need of treatment (Joint Civil Society Monitoring Forum, 2005). In other words, only 36 percent are accessing treatment.

How did it come to pass that a state seemingly so well equipped in comparison to all other African states has been outperformed by many of them? Well, although AIDS may be perceived as an exceptional issue, especially in terms of its cultural politics, the political culture surrounding AIDS treatment is also deeply influential in this and other areas of service delivery in South Africa. We will see that countrywide protests over service delivery are illustrative of deep-seated concerns over the direction of the country's development path. In relation, there are issues about the erosion of citizen leverage over services, including access to ARVs. But regarding AIDS policy itself, explanations have been many and varied, adding nuanced reflections. This chapter proffers its own explanations for the fragmented and denialist responses. It does so by locating the struggle over treatment within the broader politics of post-apartheid nation-building in tandem with the political character of the state.

AIDS, Nation-building, and Medication

AIDS, like in many other countries, has acted as a political and cultural fault line exposing tectonic plate-like ideological differences in belief, especially in attitudes toward sexuality and illness (Posel 2005). Critically, for South Africa, AIDS has also sharpened the issue of the nature and style of how a country should be governed. And the inflection given to governance has been to cast the post-apartheid state in the imagery of a continental project centered upon "African Renaissance." For Thabo Mbeki, who presided over the most fraught and fragmented period of AIDS policy responses, the image of African Renaissance was a laudable developmental and psychological initiative to return self-respect back to Africa. The problem is that as important and well intended as this initiative undoubtedly was, the African Renaissance crashed into the juggernaut of the AIDS epidemic. The pivotal issue became whether state leaders could turn the terrible collision into something to mobilize society and embolden the democratic vision of the renaissance as the basis for confronting the epidemic. As suggested, and as with the usual meticulous precision of Edwin Cameron's observations, the epidemic has always been about far more than biology and organisms (Cameron 2005). Historically, AIDS has been associated with prior cultural understandings of what induces vulnerability to disease. State leader responses to the epidemic, whether the aloofness that characterized the end period of the Mbeki era and, especially, his previously outspoken denialist stance, policy considerations are also inseparable from cultural understandings.

And those cultural understandings have been inescapably influenced by the racist context of apartheid South Africa. In particular, the chemical warfare program of the late apartheid era provided fertile ground for conspiracy theories to flourish. Evidence emerged in the 1990s that this program had been used to kill and maim black opposition figures. AIDS itself became associated with similar racial motivations, allegedly to reduce the black population. And AIDS prevention was therefore considered to be about controlling black sexuality and reproduction for sinister ends. In other words, what the national discourse on AIDS actually does is to dredge unconscious experiences and highly sensitive issues about race, sex, and disease to the surface of the nation's psyche (Fassin 2007).[2] While these experiences are particularly painful and acute, it is important to note that such interpretations of the epidemic are far from confined to South Africa.

A day after she received the Nobel Prize, Wangiri Maathi, for example, claimed in a speech in Kenya that, "Aids are not a curse from God to Africans or the Black people. It is a tool to control them designed by some evil-minded scientists."[3] In the same speech, biological warfare programs in "developed" countries were identified as responsible for the AIDS virus. Similarly, during some fieldwork in Zambia, it was not uncommon to encounter comments from people living with AIDS that they had initially believed "whites" had created AIDS (Jones 2007). And this perception had transferred to AIDS treatment, with some mentioning how they thought "ARVs bring whites." In this context, a mother told me about how her distrust of ARVs had led her and her husband to withhold treatment from their sick daughter in preference to traditional remedies. Shortly afterwards, the child died.

But in a cruel chronological twist of fate, South Africa was only just beginning to emerge from racial oppression at the same time as the epidemic began to snowball. This meant that such racialized interpretations of AIDS were only becoming more amplified. Of course, this did not have to be the case. Other paths existed, ones that sought instead to affirm active citizenship and democratization of scientific knowledge (see "Contestations and Court Cases" section of this chapter) in the context of AIDS (Robins 2005). Even these alternative routes, however, must negotiate that, whether in fact driven by cultural elites or by local cultural entrepreneurs, the HIV/AIDS crisis be read as "expressive of deeper challenges to African identity, culture and self-respect."(Kårsholm, 2006). An array of cultural practices, some newly invented, others representing something of a "comeback"—like the practice of virginity-testing—clash uneasily with more overtly liberal human rights discourses in South Africa (Vincent 2006 and see Chapter 2). And these impulses are strong and popular in many quarters.

Perhaps a common element is the need to exert some semblance of explanation, meaning, or control amidst a catastrophe such as AIDS. How else do we explain the fact that as deputy president, Mbeki felt so strongly about tackling the epidemic at one point that he enthusiastically promoted the *Virodene* project?[4] Why should he be so proactive in supporting that and not ARVs? Was this because it was represented as an African "homegrown" treatment for AIDS and stood for something that "Western" ARVs purportedly did not? This and other early post-apartheid AIDS policy fiascos, with the resultant criticism directed at the state, however, needled an already insecure government into seeking to reaffirm its control and ownership of the AIDS policy environment. Misplaced, certainly. But, nonetheless, even these misplaced responses illustrate an agency—a reaction to something, to perceived threats directed at black Africans and the sovereignty of a newly liberated South African state.

The key point is that no lesser figure than Thabo Mbeki, as president, and key allies in the ruling ANC party, sought to carve out an elitist cultural—or perhaps, more accurately, racial—position from this landscape of AIDS interventions. The tragedy for South Africa is that rather than going down the renaissance road that affirmed good governance, rights-based principles and self-respect, a diversion was made. State responses were instead taken down the slippery and treacherous path, refuting these principles and, indeed, the conventional science of AIDS. In this, it appears that the elitist discourse strives to react to what are depicted as damaging, essentializing racial slurs against African sexuality in particular. It is undeniable that much previous "Western" scientific understanding of what induces vulnerability to the disease included a prescribed pathology of certain groups, particularly concerning sexuality. But this has also been directed as much inwards to marginalized groups within the "West" as it was outwards toward non-Western areas (Stoller 1998).

On a much larger scale, Africa was often, and sometimes still is, depicted as the "other" in terms of HIV/AIDS (Jarosz 1992). For almost as long as the epidemic itself, assumed evidence of abnormal behavior and inherent practices, although usually unverified, have been taken as "scientific" explanation for Africa's status as the cradle of HIV/AIDS. Certainly, earlier discourses on vulnerability to HIV/AIDS were characterized by racist representations of the continent. But HIV/AIDS' ability to exacerbate existing stigmatization and exclusion directed at the less powerful, or so-called deviant groups and individuals, is clearly not confined to "Western" actors. Furthermore, most of this rights-based discourse has off-loaded its more overt racism. Mbali therefore makes the important point that some African state policies on HIV/AIDS, especially in South Africa, have been driven by a degree of overreaction to the more outlandish colonial, late apartheid, and racist discourses associated with the epidemic early on (Mbali 2004).

I suggested earlier that to fully comprehend both donor and African state responses, it would be useful to position them within a "geopolitics of AIDS." Previous international donor and so-called developed state inaction on supporting ARVs in the Global South, for example, can be partly explained in terms of continuations with older representations of Africa as the "other." Western donor policy was enthralled to poorly conceived prevention programs for so long. I have shown in other work how representations of Africa tended to gaze upon the continent in such a way as to rationalize inaction on providing treatment. Some of these representations depicted the continent as too devoid of sophistication, totally lacking in capacity to deliver treatment, and overall, too poor to consider technologically advanced and expensive treatment. It is with massive—yet, ultimately disastrous—irony, therefore, to observe how, in failing to respond to demands for treatment, an ANC-elite discourse itself essentialized treatment as "Western," and HIV/AIDS as related only to "structural poverty." For too long, this strand of the ANC discourse has been stuck in a bizarre and deadly waltz. It is a waltz that rejects, but also must embrace, the flip side of its own binary opposite: the "West" and "underdevelopment." This reaction was simply not needed given that HIV/AIDS discourse and its science has undoubtedly been modified. Tremendous efforts have been made to insert a human rights focus and also important corrective social, economic, and political factors in understanding the epidemic in Africa.[5] Uncovering the reasons for President Mbeki's denialist position and the refusal to acknowledge the link between HIV as leading to AIDS would involve a book in itself (see Fassin 2007). Some of the reasons already mentioned are elaborated upon further because they are directly relevant for the discussion that follows about ARV treatment in South Africa.

A fascinating window on the ANC HIV/AIDS discourse can be gleaned, for example, from a cursory reading of the now infamous position paper issued early in 2002.[6] The paper, entitled *Cato Hlongwane, caravans, cats, geese, foot & mouth statistics: HIV/AIDS and the struggle for humanisation of the African* is said to be authored by Peter Mokaba, with contributions by Mbeki rumored but unsubstantiated. Mokaba was a leading ANC figure who himself was a bitter denialist, even as the disease was ravaging his own body and eventually killed him. The paper rages powerfully against what it depicts as Western biomedical stigmatization of African sexuality. The continent, it suggests, is represented as a repository of degeneration with "behaviour of our people . . . pre-prescribed by the scientists of the developed world" (p. 103) through "a campaign whose result is further to entrench their dehumanization" (p. 5). There are crosscutting discourses that squarely situate the continent's vulnerability in terms of externally generated underdevelopment and poverty rather than "self-inflicted" behavior:

> In spite of our friends, the friends of Africa, we must stand up to say that we have had enough of the insults that demean Africans, whatever their nationality. The time has come that we gather the courage and intellect to say that we too are human, as human as any other human being. We are neither freaks, nor do we behave like freaks. We have never been barbarians and are not now. We are poor. We live in conditions of under-development. We are concentrated within the tropics and suffer from and enjoy the physical conditions that nature has imposed on this part of the globe. None of this makes us sub-human. Nor should the impact of disease, including AIDS, that afflicts us, be used in the name of questionable science and friendship with us, to reduce us to a peculiar species of humanity likely to slip back into a state of savagery (p. 128).

AIDS is represented as a syndrome rather than a disease, implying that people do not actually die of AIDS but poverty and the opportunistic infections it nurtures. Overall, the defense of the dissident position on AIDS is to pit itself against racism in the orthodox/conventional position. "Even the story of HIV developed in a very racist way," we are told by Mokaba. To depict AIDS as a sexually transmitted disease is somehow to reinforce the dehumanization.[7]

It is particularly relevant for the book to note how this discourse has had serious implications for the role of treatment for HIV/AIDS. ARVs became pivotal to the Mokaba/Mbeki-inspired ideological tussle against Western biomedicine and racism. In the *Castro Hlongwane* document, the pharmaceutical industry is depicted as propagating false information on HIV/AIDS in order to sell its drugs.[8] Those who promote the "orthodox" argument that HIV leads to AIDS and that it can be controlled by ARVs, again, are depicted as reinforcing the colonial dehumanization of the African. Indeed, these antiretrovirals are labeled as highly toxic, and even as responsible for death, due to side-effects. As an apparent medical solution to HIV/AIDS, treatment is forcefully rejected as "Western" medicalizing of the real issues—"poverty" and "underdevelopment." ARVs are perceived to not attack the underlying cause of immune suppression and offer little, if no, hope.[9] That these ideas have had such influence on the direction of post-apartheid AIDS policy has baffled and disappointed many in equal measure. But to fully understand how these ideas could gain such influence also requires insight into the political character of the post-apartheid state.

Political Characteristics and Responses to AIDS

Interest in the relationship between HIV/AIDS and governance initially tended to examine how AIDS erodes governments and formal democratic capacity.[10] More recently, notable exceptions highlight one or more political components of it that *shape* policy frameworks and responses.[11] Level of capacity in the health sector, composition of the bureaucracy, and leadership style are some issues, for example, cited by Parkhurst and Lush to explain the very different responses to AIDS in South Africa and Uganda. Putzel identifies a number of dimensions in explaining President Museveni of Uganda's particularly open and proactive stance on AIDS (Putzel 2003a). Some of these impulses stem from the leader's openness to scientific evidence. It is revealing to note, for instance, that once Museveni removed expatriates from several key scientific posts and replaced them with Ugandans, this appeared to facilitate trust of science. But there were other factors, such as national security (see under further discussion of Uganda).

One of the most advanced analyses to date is provided by Patterson (2006), who seeks to locate state responses within a broader understanding of the nature of the state. In this, she identifies four key characteristics of the state in Africa that are considered to have a critical bearing upon AIDS policies: the degree of *centralization* (in terms of the degree of executive and presidential power); the degree of *neo-patrimonialism* (at a basic level of definition, corruption); the degree of *security* (political stability); and, overall, the degree of state *capacity* (measured crudely in terms of gross national product). These characteristics are used as a foil against which to measure AIDS policy responses. So, for example, whereas one would expect, on the basis of these characteristics, that a middle income country like South Africa performs well in terms of their "AIDS Program Effort" in comparison to most other African countries, it is apparently outperformed by Uganda, and more so by Rwanda.[12] Patterson's findings are useful in problematizing explanations of AIDS policy and programs. She brings into focus the critical role of power, representation, and political institutions in understanding responses to the epidemic. In particular, she suggests that despite the low levels of neo-patrimonialism and centralization in South Africa, AIDS policy has in fact been an exception in experiencing a much higher level of centralization. Political characteristics of the state enabled the particular stance presented by Mbeki and others to become manifest in the fabric of its institutions. In so doing, executive control of institutional structures undermined the potential for transparency, multisectoral mobilization, and steering of responses. Take the South African National AIDS Council (SANAC) as an example. Until very recently, whereas representatives from the government sector (sixteen in total) dominated SANAC, there was only one NGO representative to represent the 600-plus organizations involved with HIV/AIDS (van Der Vliet 2004, 58). Scientists and researchers were not recognized as a sector and were therefore not represented, while traditional healers were the only representatives from the medical profession.[13] Notable oppositional civil society organizations, such as the Treatment Action Campaign, were also excluded. It does, however, finally look like this is changing following the change in presidency, with a broadening of political space for civil society inclusion in AIDS policymaking.

In terms of leadership, one of the biggest motivations for the proactive stance taken in Uganda appears to be concerns over security and the threat posed by AIDS to Museveni's armed forces (he had been leader of the National Resistance Movement). De Waal also suggests, as mentioned in the introduction, the political function and benefits of adopting such a stance to enhance Uganda's international reputation with donors, amongst others. In contrast, from 1994, the newly elected ANC lacked such urgency on AIDS. The new government was more preoccupied with racial reconciliation and democratic and economic stability and transformation than with AIDS. Another factor concerns the influence of a popularly elected political party credited with liberation. Without any significant challenge from discredited, and small opposition parties, the ANC nonetheless felt it imperative to imprint party loyalty upon its members. The AIDS response reveals that such loyalty has been to the cost of discouraging internal dissent (see "Contestations and Court Cases" section of this chapter). Party loyalty has been paramount, hindering both the capacity and independence of the civil service in South Africa to respond to AIDS (Heywood 2003). Rather than creating an independent civil service that caters to the needs of the population, these ends have been subordinated to serving party loyalty. So while levels of neopatrimonialism, according to Patterson, appear low—and it would be interesting to get more recent figures for this and particularly to look at specific measurements—arguably, the party structure acts as a vehicle for patronage in terms of promotion, political favor, or otherwise. Contrary to Patterson's findings, there is mounting evidence in South Africa of the substantial economic benefits accrued as dominant party, and hence state patronage machinery, positions increasingly overlap with access to economic resources (see Chapter 3). Evidence for this can be partly gauged in the context of service delivery riots (see "South Africa's Development Path, Service Delivery, and Protest" section in this chapter). In a sense related to these riots, while significant financial commitment has been made by the state to AIDS, as with other services, capacity issues continue to hinder delivery.

In the face of significant skepticism and opposition to ARVs from government, and in the absence of a viable political opposition party, a significant force for change has come from civil society. The latter, in conjunction with the use of constitutional human rights and the courts, has been a very effective political source in contesting state AIDS policy responses.

Contestations and Court Cases

In affirming the constitutional duty of the state toward respecting, protecting, and promoting the right to access health care, one particular high-profile court case (*Minister of Health v TAC* 2002) in the process exposed the contested claims made over ARVs in South Africa. Since 1999, the Treatment Action Campaign, the leading AIDS civil society organization, had made repeated requests that the government accelerate its policy on prevention of mother-to-child transmission of HIV/AIDS (or "MTCT," which takes place from the infected mother to child either during pregnancy, birth, and/or breast-feeding). The government refused to accelerate its program but following a meeting in 2000, decided that MTCT policy would be focused upon two test sites in each province. Critically, it was decided that provision of the drug Nevirapine—central to preventing transmission to the child—would be limited to these sites (eighteen in total). The applicants took issue with the government program restricting the provision of the drug to the designated sites. The second major complaint was that in restricting policy, the government did not have sufficient planning for a national program to progressively realize the access over time. These restrictions were deemed unreasonable by the applicants in view of the state's constitutional obligations to provide access to health care for people living with HIV/AIDS and in what actions it was taking to prevent MTCT. TAC took the government to the high court and, upon losing, the government's appeal in the Constitutional Court in 2002 reflects a fascinating public scrutiny of state policy on ARVs.

There, before court, in the eyes of the South African and world media glare, the crux of the issue considered by the court was whether the government's policy could be considered "reasonable." Government argued that it wanted to develop and monitor its human and material resources for delivery of a complete package including testing and counseling, dispensing of Nevirapine, and the provision of follow-up services to pregnant women (such as availability of bottle-feeding, where this had to be substituted for breast-feeding). The overall defense concerned the need for appropriate methods and procedures regarding implementation, cultural problems related to bottle-feeding, and absence of clean water for the latter. The government argued that capacity did not exist and would be costly to expand. In addition, the government case emphasized questions about the *safety of the drug and also the underlying conditions of poverty* in the country. Increased risks associated with the drug were suggested where children were growing up with inadequate nutrition and sanitation. The latter reasoning, particularly the linking of the safety of the drug to environmental and material factors, was a clear indication of the skeptical denialist views that had been driving government policy on treatment and that surfaced in the Cato

Hlongwane document. The reasons Africans get infected, so the argument of the earlier section goes, is a product of structural factors, and if the link between HIV and AIDS is denied, then medication, such as that used for preventing MTCT, is superfluous and even harmful and toxic.

The court, however, stressed that "courts may—and if need be must—use their wide powers to make orders that affect policy as well as legislation" (Minister of Health v TAC p. 64). A guiding consideration in the court's reasoning was that "policy is and should be flexible. It may be changed at any time and the court is always free to change policies where it considers it appropriate to do so." It therefore followed that lifting the restrictions "to make nevirapine available at all state hospitals and clinics where there are testing and counselling facilities that will call for a change in policy." Cost was not considered to be a determining factor because there was already existing capacity beyond the test sites and the drug had been donated to the government for free. Extra training for counseling was also considered to be quick and relatively cheap. The court found existing policy unreasonable and declared: "Once the restriction is removed, government will be able to devise and implement a more comprehensive policy that will give access to health care services to HIV-positive mothers and their newborn children, and include the administration of Nevirapine where that is appropriate. Policy as reformulated must meet the constitutional requirement of providing reasonable measures within available resources for the progressive realisation of the rights of such women and newborn children" (p. 68). The court's interpretation therefore resonated with key rights-based principles surrounding health and treatment (see Chapter 2 for more detail). These principles foreground accessibility and equality of access and mapping out the corresponding obligations. The obligations concerned removing obstacles (negative obligations), as well as the need to take positive measures (active steps, such as extending counseling, etc.) in order to fulfill the right of access to health care. Furthermore, in a damning view of the lack of multisectoral collaboration that had characterized responses to AIDS in South Africa, the court also requested that greater transparency was required and "regretted" that no program had been disclosed by six (all then ANC-led) of nine provincial health ministers. Indeed, to illustrate the grip of party loyalty upon national and provincial administrations, in reviewing affidavit material submitted to the court, Heywood (2003) noticed how each provincial submission had one particular spelling error exactly the same. This appears to reflect the level of centralized executive interference in AIDS policy.

The court therefore found the policy to be unreasonable as it "excludes those who could be reasonably included" and called for the immediate lifting on restrictions so that whilst not everyone could immediately claim the right, progressive realization (such as planning) was the guiding principle with the goal of access to all. Government policy and, by implication, the judgment of key figures within it had been openly questioned in public and ordered by the court to be changed. Such was the highly charged backdrop to access to ARVs in South Africa. Following this court ruling, and with concerted international and national momentum for treatment as well as internal divisions within the ruling party and cabinet, came the apparent government U-turn on treatment. But negative attitudes continued. In 2003, for example, minister of finance, Trevor Manuel, announced his 2003 budget speech, with over R3 billion allocated for HIV/AIDS. Shortly after, however, he was quoted as describing—somewhat tellingly—ARVs as akin to '"Western voodoo." These statements resonated with the more public views of the minister of health and Mbeki himself. As one example, at the end of 2004, in the online publication *ANC Today*, which includes a weekly "letter from the president," an article on Nevirapine used very strong imagery of Africans treated as if they were "guinea pigs." One particular U.S. research institute is described—inaccurately—as having "entered into a conspiracy with a pharmaceutical company to tell lies to promote the sales of nevirapine in Africa, with absolutely no consideration of the health impact of those lies on the lives of millions of Africans" (ANC 2004). Again, conspiracy, drugs, and depiction of Africans as exploited reflects use of those key discursive tropes identified earlier in this chapter. Also, in an effort to discredit opposition to the government's stance, the same article claims that the "central mission" of the TAC "is to guarantee and improve the sale of anti-retroviral drugs."[14] The deadly waltz continued its dance. The space for ARVs is effectively closed down and room for political maneuvers is also hamstrung. The power of the discourse is to condemn and demote ARVs as "unAfrican," "anti-African," or "Western." There are numerous other examples. And these refutations therefore beg the question of what, then, are deemed to be African alternatives.

"African Alternatives"

"I was discussing with the complainant telling her that I have heard that there was a certain woman, I told her that a comrade of mine had learned that there was a certain woman who would mix these herbs that would help in this disease. I told her about actually two people, one in KwaZulu-Natal and the one locally here, that they help people with those herbs. I said this in order to encourage her to take those herbs if she wanted to and maybe she could be helped." (State and Jacob Zuma 2006:937).[15] "He [Zuma] said a comrade he trusted very much had come to him and recommended these herbs, which were put together by as certain healer. He said perhaps these herbs could help bring my

CD4 count up . . . [and that another herb] being tested in KwaZulu-Natal hospitals [could] . . . perhaps be a cure for me" (Complainant 2006).[16]

South Africa has, for ten years, been acquainted with key leaders who have been skeptical of ARVs. When she was health minister, Manto Tshabalala-Msimang, in particular, stated on many occasions that the African potato, olive oil, lemon juice, and garlic, on the one hand, and traditional medication on the other, are more appropriate "African alternatives" to ARVs. Her preference has been to focus on the role of such alternatives in boosting the immune system. And, furthermore, important debates on the role of nutrition in also benefiting the immune system have ended upon being stripped of their significance. Instead, they are shoehorned into the tight fitting binary opposition and can only be understood in opposition to ARVs. In talking about traditional medication, for example, Tshabalala-Msimang says that it has "been used by our people long before the advent . . . of other forms of medicine. And our people still use traditional medicine even today . . . and you can't stop them from using traditional medicines."[17] While patently accurate to describe the widespread use and appeal of traditional medication in contemporary South Africa, as underscored in the above statements by Zuma and the Complainant in his rape trial (and see especially Chapter 6), the phrasing "long before the advent of other forms of medicine"—such as ARVs—is very revealing. Traditional medicine has also been placed in binary opposition to ARVs; it is ascribed with properties more African in nature, something timeless and affirmative of African identity. It is African and ARVs are not. The minister's predilection for promoting apparent "African alternatives" to ARVs results in it getting its own chapter in the comprehensive plan. This is often in stark contrast to the treatment literature produced by the minister's own department of health (in partnership with other organizations). It states, quite clearly, in some of this educative literature that traditional medicines—for example, including the African potato—mean that: "If you take them when you take ART, the treatment may not work."[18]

There is a national discourse taking place on the role of ARVs and alternative, or complementary, treatment of AIDS. This permeates from the upper echelons of state and to the local *Shabeen*. In 2006, the sensational court case concerning rape allegations against Jacob Zuma, since elected leader of the ANC, captured the imagination of the country for many reasons. Amidst all the more controversial statements—about political conspiracy, Zuma's comments about AIDS prevention, and the aggressive form of questioning of the complainant—less visible but also present was discussion of treatment for AIDS. The two statements at the start of this section indicate that there was discussion of traditional herbs during the trial. The HIV positive complainant suggested Zuma promoted the role of herbs to better her condition. The prosecution engineered the exchange in order to try and prove that Zuma did not use a condom, either because he was allegedly already HIV-positive (and hence, they implied, his knowledgeable discussion of herbs somehow showed this) or because there was no consent (implying that rape took place). Although both claims were proven to be lacking any basis, the exchange did nonetheless confirm that there was a discussion about the merits of traditional medication. And, although Zuma's own testimony falls short of suggesting these may represent a cure—and in fact his full account situates traditional medication as one of many approaches to the epidemic—it does indicate belief in traditional medication as beneficial in treating AIDS and that the complainant was encouraged to pursue this. Unlike the minister of health, who, for many years, has portrayed alternatives to ARVs, we certainly should not read into Zuma's account that these traditional herbs represent, for him, an alternative to the exclusion of ARVs. It tends, rather, to demonstrate that there is a multilayered discourse taking place on treatment that reveals itself in the Zuma "rape case." The point is that whilst statements made by Thabo Mbeki, the minister of health, and many others are criticized, we should not ignore that competing views of AIDS treatment are more widespread, subtle, and can also coexist with, or reject, ARVs (see Chapter 6).

The death of the popular HIV-positive DJ, Khabzela, and his rejection of ARVs were mentioned in the introduction to this book. Furthermore, soon after, another high-profile death involved that of Nozipho Bhengu, the daughter of a former ANC MP, Ruth Bhengu. Like Khabzela, Nozipho's decision to publicly disclose her status was lauded as a very brave decision in the face of continuing stigma surrounding HIV and AIDS. Then, like Khabzela, she rejected ARVs, with her mother claiming they had worsened her condition. Also, like Khabzela, Nozipho initially suggested the benefits of taking Tine van der Maas' diet of lemon, garlic, olive oil, and *Africa's solution*. The TAC suggested that both Khabzela and Bhengu were pressured by the denialist winds blowing around South Africa. Indeed, there is an official "denialist" position from within sections of the state. But we should not be blinded to how this feeds *into* and also *from* broader collective and individual responses to the epidemic and especially perceptions of ARVs (see chapters 5 and 6).

The power of AIDS discourse has also undoubtedly conditioned state-civil society relations. There is substantial evidence to suggest that government has colluded with certain actors to promote their agenda surrounding so-called alternative treatments. As one example, multivitamin company owner Matthias Rath apparently gained preferential treatment to import his unregistered vitamin products into South Africa to conduct experiments in a local community in Khayelitsha Township, and he also spread misinformation through media advertisements. Both he and the Traditional Healers' Organisation were indicted by the Cape High Court for making statements alleging improper connections, again, between the TAC and, in what is a recurring pattern, the pharmaceutical industry, whose interests they said the TAC represented. The minister of health has sought to build alliances with more compliant civil society organizations, such as the National Association of People with AIDS, in order to sideline those more critical of government's response to the epidemic. There is evidence suggesting that Rath's money has been used to underpin many such related activities, even implicating the Medical Research Council itself.

Key leading political figures have certainly legitimized denialist debate. Credibility has been lent to popular forms of AIDS denial and to undermine established scientific "truths" concerning the epidemic. An intriguing issue is to what extent this denialist discourse has influenced public knowledge and attitudes for the majority of South Africans not exposed to scientific debate (Robins 2004). Another is how it has been lent to the promotion not only of alternative treatments but also traditional practices. One more is the considerable impact upon opportunities for marketing for sale unregulated and unproven "alternative" products. A cursory read of the classified section of popular newspapers, like the tabloid *Sun*, for example, at any one time, reveals that many herbalists advertise—sometimes as many as nine times per issue—and proclaim to cure all kinds of diseases. One healer even claims, "He will heal your illness and related disease, like HIV-related disease . . ."[19] A huge issue, therefore, and one explored in chapters 5 and 6, concerns popular perceptions of ARVs and also the role of alternative and traditional explanations of and treatments for AIDS.

The outcome, as suggested, has been, for a long time, uncannily similar to Western donors: until relatively recently, the South African government and Western donors alike had arrested the chances of poor people's access to lifesaving treatment. These racial fault lines associated with HIV/AIDS and the issue of treatment show up again and again. These damaging statements and views continue to be embedded in public discourse and attitudes. The slow pace of rollout also appears correlated to the often-contradictory comments from the minister of health as well as the withdrawal of Mbeki from speaking publicly on the issue at all.

Another facet is how the lingering presence of denialism serves to impact upon levels of personal denial. Further evidence of government skepticism, for example, was apparent in 2006 in the context of another court case, this time involving the right of prisoners to access ARVs. The government had obstructed an interim court order to enable access of prisoners in need of ARVs. This prompted the AIDS Law Project, a nongovernmental organization, acting on behalf of the PLWA prisoners, to state: "[T]he real issue at stake is the failure of government to lead on HIV/AIDS, to comply with a duty of care to people in need of health services including those who need antiretroviral therapy. Instead, the government uses this "blood relationship" to disguise its callous AIDS denialism, bureaucratic obstructionism and disregard for the right to life of people living with HIV/AIDS. If government had a real case, it would not undermine the judiciary."[20] In 2006, the mounting frustration and criticism against the government culminated in widespread condemnation of the minister of health at the International HIV/AIDS Conference in Toronto. This was precipitated by Tshabalala-Msimang's exhibition at the conference, which promoted beetroot and alternative treatments for AIDS while downgrading and even initially excluding any role for ARVs. Many observers regarded this as perhaps the zenith of deliberate and public attempts to undermine the role of ARVs in treating people with AIDS. Some newspapers publicly called for the minister's dismissal.[21]

The frustration with the slow pace of delivery of ARVs and difficulty of ensuring accountability obviously reflects a distinct ideological tussle surrounding AIDS. But given the political characteristics mentioned, the lack of delivery does tend to mirror more general problems in service delivery throughout South Africa. Service delivery problems are discussed in some detail because they reflect an important backdrop to the more detailed local analysis to come in subsequent chapters.

South Africa's Development Path, Service Delivery, and Protest

"The council thinks that because we are poor and live in underprivileged areas they do not have to provide us with running water and electricity. They think because we are poor we do not deserve the same rights as the rich and they do not have to deliver on the promises made to us" (Community Representative, Soshanguve).[22]

Since 1994, a major policy consideration of successive governments has been to bring about social transformation of public services in South Africa. In this task of realigning, rationalizing, extending, and financing public services, there is now unprecedented budgetary support of around 60 percent of the total budget for social services sectors—education, health, welfare, and social services (Fakir 2007). Yet, for all this, which Fakir, amongst others, calls a remarkable achievement, the question posed is why do such levels of poverty and inequality persist and, above all, why does widespread dissatisfaction about public service remain? A fundamental consideration is therefore citizens' own experiences of service delivery. After all, as various commentators allude to, it is through service delivery institutions such as hospitals, schools, and home affairs offices that citizens experience public services. According to Ngema, such service points are

> often run down, visibly dirty, have shortages of staff, equipment and vehicles, have no proper signage and seating areas for citizens, have no rest areas or other facilities for staff, struggle to provide clean reliable water and other basic services, and are poorly managed and unsupported by other senior echelons in the management hierarchy. [It is also most frequently the point at which citizens experience corrupt or inept officials or public servants who simply don't do what they're supposed to]. It is quite clear that the public service has not fully internalised the critical role that service points play in the service delivery value chain, and as the 'moments of truth' as far as citizens are concerned serves to undermine and render irrelevant everything that may be otherwise soundly managed and executed.[23]

These "moments of truth" are beginning to impact not only developmental but also political stability in South Africa. In 2005, the minister of safety and security reported, for example, that across South Africa, a total of 881 illegal and 5,085 legal protests took place (Atkinson 2007:58). Most of these protests are directly related to community frustration over poor service delivery and, arguably, their alienation from mainstream representative democracy (and the more formal participatory channels associated with "specialist" legislative or party political public hearings). Protests continue to rock the country and appear correlated, according to Atkinson, to three particular characteristics.

First, they tend to be areas characterized by poor service delivery, involving delays and operational problems. This is often related to the chronic shortage of qualified staff to implement service delivery, particularly municipal engineers. In terms of housing, for example, since 1994, 1.8 million subsidized houses have been provided. Despite government figures that 200,000 houses are being provided each year, the backlog in 2006 was placed at 2.4 million. Government has said itself that at this pace, the "*millennium development goal*" housing target will not be met. This mismatch in demand and supply is reflected in an upward trend in growth of informal settlements and homelessness and an intensifying pace of evictions and land invasions.

Second, these areas also have limited channels for residents to voice their concerns. The protests, although manifesting frustrations over living conditions, may therefore pose a potentially dangerous challenge to democratic stability in South Africa. In this, the minister for housing recently highlighted the potential for even greater instability in the run-up to the 2009 general elections: "Inadequacies in the delivery of basic services continue to be our biggest threat in the consolidation of democracy" (Minister for Housing Lindiwe Sisulu, speaking at the ANC's National Executive Committee's *lekgotla*).[24]

People are beginning to feel disillusioned with the democratic dispensation that is failing to raise the standard of living for most of the population and that does not appear to reduce inequality. Such a dynamic may also be feeding the growth of populism surrounding former state deputy president Jacob Zuma, who, in late 2007, was elected president of the ANC. A correlation can certainly be made between Zuma's growth in support, with his victory as the president of ANC and the drawing to the end the Mbeki era. In the final weeks of the Mbeki presidency, the following characteristics appear, if anything, to be amplified: "The closing down of space for open, robust, debate within the ANC more generally not just on the left—[which] has driven too many in the party, and the alliance, into Zuma's demagogic arms."[25]

The quotation at the start of this section by a resident in Soshanguve, near Temba/Hammanskraal captures the sense of frustration detailed in later chapters that exists in many communities. There are strong feelings that promises made by government have been broken. In this area, rioters barricaded parts of the township and destroyed public property following violent clashes with police and residents. Police, using rubber bullets, shot several residents, and several policemen were injured in the clashes. Residents demanded that the city council develop essential services and fulfill its promises after thirteen years, according to the representative quoted above. The council responded that they had not been able to develop the land in question because of budgetary constraints, which, after the riots, were apparently lifted. Most damaging, as also evidenced by the quotation, is the sense in which the human rights edifice carved out in the post-apartheid era is somehow deemed only accessible to the "rich" as opposed to the "poor" communities. With notable exceptions, whether the promise of rights is keeping up with the pace of increasing developmental needs remains doubtful (Jones and Stokke 2005).

Third, residents in these areas may be more likely to perceive local government as corrupt. This might include increased salaries and expenditure upon administration that appears unjust and that may constitute the fuse igniting many of these protests. It is also an issue of concern duly acknowledged by government. The government took the positive step of launching the Local Government Anti-corruption Strategy, modeled on the Public Service Anti-corruption Strategy. Renewed efforts are being made to instill a culture of intolerance toward corruption. Minister of Local and Provincial Government Sydney Mufumadi, refreshingly, conceded that corruption at the local level is so serious that it threatens service delivery and is responsible for failures in the latter. But how this is applied will remain key to whether it is merely good policy or effectively implemented. Other examples of attempts to respond to growing corruption at a national level were the ANC's formation of a high level task team, resulting in a policy document entitled, "Revolutionary Morality: The ANC and Business." It contained interesting examples and insights into the impact of business in contributing to unethical behavior and acknowledged that, to date, attempts have failed "in taming the beast of unethical behavior in our ranks." The impression, however, is nonetheless of a failure to tackle this other than in discussion and with some recommendations, which are unlikely to have much of an impact. The code of ethics and the ministerial handbook appear inadequate to stem the tide of corrupt, or at least unethical, practices whereby politicians, ministers, and so on, have business interests. But what is as damaging is the lack of a broader public debate on these issues. Rather than making denials, a frank and open debate about the desirability of mixing business interests and political roles is urgently required.

Service delivery in South Africa is therefore confronted by a series of challenges. As summarized by Fakir (2007), these include institutional weaknesses; poor human resource management; lack of planning and development; widespread gaps in the quality and relevance of training and institutions; poor linkages and partnerships between government and training providers; an inadequate focus on norms, values, attitudes, and orientation of public officials; a lack of credible data; and limited capacity for basic analysis and planning. To this should be added the urgent need for an impetus towards building greater responsiveness and accountability of service providers to the executive, the public and stronger political oversight.

Contrary to enabling greater interface between service providers and the public, the Mbeki era has also been associated with a growing and disturbing trend whereby police used disproportionate force against protestors. The right to demonstrate is increasingly outlawed. High-profile incidents include *Abahlali base Mjondolo*, a shack-dwellers organization whose leaders were beaten by police outside Durban. In relation to this, when a recent spontaneous march to the police station took place, where the leaders were held, police opened fire (including use of live ammunition) without any apparent warning, citing that the march was an illegal gathering. The Freedom of Expression Institute (FXI) deemed this an unconstitutional and illegal response. Police should have attempted to negotiate, give warnings, and only used firearms under strict conditions.

In another incident in February 2006, police raided informal settlements in Durban, arresting and, it is alleged, severely beating some residents who, again, represented *Abahlali*. The latter had wanted to protest over poor housing delivery. According to the FXI, the movement in question had notified the local authorities that they planned to march. It was therefore entirely legal according to the *Regulation of Gatherings Act*. Taking place just two days prior to the local elections, the raids by police on the communities in question appeared to be a preemptive action instigated at the request of the city manager. According to the FXI, it represents "an extremely dangerous precedent for our legal system" and that "such high-handed police action is completely out of tune with a democratic society and is, rather, reminiscent of the days of Apartheid. We want to remind the eThekwini Metro Police that their ongoing actions in various Durban shack settlements are illegal and unconstitutional."[26] These disproportionate and illegal responses reflect the continuing downgrading and delegitimization of forms of protest that exist outside of formal party politics.

Furthermore, the Orange Farm Water Crisis Committee was involved in another incident whereby police opened fire, apparently without warning, although some press reports do indicate that police attempted negotiations. At any rate, the shooting was indiscriminate, injuring many people nearby who were not part of the demonstration. One of the officials from the South African Transport and Allied Workers Union was shot and seriously wounded by police without any apparent justification.

In 2005, service delivery protest and frustrations over limited access to ARVs overlapped. In the Eastern Cape city of Queenstown, local members of the Treatment Action Campaign demonstrated about the lack of progress on access to antiretroviral treatment for HIV/AIDS in the province. Then, apparently without warning, police assaulted the protestors and opened fire with rubber bullets and released teargas as people ran away. It was reported that forty people were injured and ten were treated for gunshot wounds, although none of the protestors was arrested or charged with any crime.[27] Human Rights Watch, who documented the incident, suggested that there was no indication that the actions by the South African police met international standards for the appropriate use of force by police. What seems to connect these and many more incidents is that they indicate that even when used in good faith, the *Regulation of Gatherings Act* prevents spontaneous gatherings due to its seven-day-notice requirement.[28] According to the Freedom of Expression Institute: "The result is a frightening environment of repression developing within South Africa, with free expression constantly being in danger—especially the free expression of poor communities for whom their main form of expression is to take to the streets."

Thus, the ability to do something about poor standards in service delivery is being restricted. These issues provide an important context within which to understand issues in the delivery of ARVs to local communities and where and whether an impetus for accountability lies and may be created. The issue of service delivery is a critical one for South Africa, and for ARV rollout itself—one that requires some insight into the state's organizational culture. That culture was graphically represented in rigid state resistance to extend access to AIDS treatment. Arguably, in the post-apartheid era, the state more generally tends to interpret popular participation either only insofar as an endorsement or, it is supportive of state policies, rather than an independent force for challenging and reorienting government policies (Jones and Stokke 2005; Greenstein 2003:15).

A New Dawn for ARV Delivery?

In 2006, during the minister of health's extended absence from office due to serious illness, there had been encouraging signs of renewed multisectoral collaboration and more genuinely inclusive policymaking.[29] The support of the then deputy president and the deputy minister of health for a consultative process surrounding the drafting of the National Strategic Plan for HIV/AIDS and STIs, as well as plans for the revitalization of the South African National AIDS Council, appeared to reflect a new dawn for cooperation between state and civil society. That said, by 2007, the apparent isolation of Deputy Minister Nozizwe Madlala-Routledge, not only from her minister but also from the Department of Health and ANC party officials, indicated that the issue was by no means resolved. Indeed, this was confirmed by the subsequent dismissal of Madlala-Routledge on somewhat spurious grounds. Although an official government reason was never given, the former deputy minister has suggested that President Mbeki cited, in a meeting, disapproval of her attendance at an international AIDS conference in Spain. However, the real reason would appear to be that Madlala-Routledge visited a state hospital in the Eastern Cape amidst hearing reports about an extremely high level of infant mortality—2,000 still births in fourteen years—in the maternity ward. Apparently shocked at the poor standards of care she saw at the Frere hospital, with chronic shortages and a very high turnover of staff and lack of equipment, Madlala-Routledge shared her alarm with the national press: "It really shows what is a national emergency in my view, particularly with infant mortality seen as an important human development indicator."[30]

Statements by the minister of health and the president himself contradicted these comments.[31] The dismissal of Madlala-Routledge therefore dealt a blow to the momentum giving new impetus toward less denialist and exclusionary AIDS and health policymaking. Other areas of continuing disputes concern government proposals for regulating medicines. Foremost amongst these—and as vindicated by Chapter 6—is that the urgent need for regulation of unproven "treatments" will instead be further weakened by government's political maneu vers. Given the support of alternative and traditional products by some members of the cabinet and their skepticism of ARVs, as documented, these are very alarming proposals. The amendments proposed by government are to the Draft Medicines and Related Substances Amendment Bill in 2008. These amendments would give the minister of health, a political appointment, greater decision-making power on approving untested products as well as powers to block registration of certain proven medicines. Because this decision-making would then be over and above the specialist technical advice of the Medicines Control Council suggests that political expediency continued to undermine independent scientific standards and regulation in South Africa (AIDS Law Project 2008).

The new dawn, if this is what we can really call it (and see Conclusion) when qualified by these ongoing disputes, however, is critical in the fight against HIV/AIDS in South Africa. Hitherto the response concerning treatment has been heavily qualified by two caveats essential for contextualizing ARV treatment in South Africa.

First, as suggested, the heavily politicized nature of AIDS has meant that debate on highly complex issues has fallen victim to deeply polarized exchanges between civil society and government, limiting debate to "either/or" positions on ARVs. Debate and discussion on issues such as public and patient perception of ARVs, patient anxiety, AIDS-related stigma, the role of nutrition, traditional and alternative medication, and health citizenship, sadly, have been underdeveloped. Similar to many countries experiencing high HIV/AIDS prevalence, the huge shortfall in people on treatment compared to those who need it in South Africa reflects a broad range of obstacles in accessing treatment that can be termed both "up-" and "down-" stream.

"Upstream," for example, may concern political and economic dynamics that certainly influence access in terms of funding, human resources needed to deliver treatment, as well as the pivotal role of political will and leadership in galvanizing responses to treatment. On another level, however, a complex set of "downstream" factors, conditioned by the interplay of local and extralocal factors, encompass access from the point of view of the individual person living with HIV/AIDS. As suggested, these "downstream" complexities have hitherto tended to be overshadowed by the contested and urgent nature of the politics involved in making treatment available in South Africa. But the issues surrounding access and, above all, in maintaining access, mean people living with AIDS must negotiate conflicting and confusing messages on ARVs. Furthermore, access to health care is governed by local knowledge and complex local geographies of institutional and social access and exclusion as much as by what national leaders do or do not do.

Second, ARV "rollout" lies alongside service delivery problems more generally in South Africa. The task of engineering the transition from apartheid-era exclusion from adequate services to instead make sure the majority benefit from inclusive provision is considerable. It also risks being dominated by approaches reifying technical issues and delivery to "passive" recipients. Whether in talking about electricity, water or housing, health services, the critical role of the nature and quality of the local interface between citizens and service providers is little emphasized. We should therefore also be asking whether there is a causal link between that organizational culture and, indeed, governance of institutions, such as hospitals, and the nature and quality of ARV delivery.

It has been suggested in the chapter that because the struggle to access treatment in South Africa has been so consuming and polarizing, more subtle issues in access have tended to be subsumed in larger political conflicts. Although changing considerably in recent years—with increasing focus upon operational issues and patient retention—it is nonetheless perhaps inevitable that access to treatment has been indelibly influenced by the broader politics of treatment in South Africa. This provides an essential backdrop to discussing, more specifically, the nature of "access" to treatment. An important starting point is to explore its definition and meaning so that we may better understand its role either in mitigating or reinscribing geographies of political and social inequality. We turn, therefore, to a discussion of the scope and nature of "access" itself and what role human rights and clinical criteria play in it.

CHAPTER 2

Conceptualizing Human Rights and "Access" to Medication

The issue of "access" to medication, and the lack of it, has long been associated with the stark inequalities characterizing the global AIDS epidemic. Although treatment has been available since the mid-1990s, this was confined to more developed countries, or, wealthier people living with AIDS in the global south who could afford it. In effect, poorer regions were priced out until recently. This disparity immediately qualifies whether something is accessible or merely available between and within countries. Human rights have played a pivotal role in galvanizing responses to correct for the lack of access. Yet, there are deep-seated tensions within human rights discourse and practice concerning whether priority should be given, first, to "freedoms" (civil and political rights) or to "freedom from want" (socioeconomic rights), and, second, how to accommodate different cultural contexts within the universal values of human rights. It is therefore of intrigue to inquire about how human rights interface and deal with issues of culture and socioeconomic and political inequality. That is, if we accept that human rights are a part of the social world we live in, and if they are to remain something other than abstract and normative principles, they require meaningful awareness of, and negotiation with, social practices.

The chapter does so by briefly looking at the contested nature of human rights and how this should be considered in rights-based approaches to AIDS-related goods, services, and information. Furthermore, specifically in the context of access to ARVs, a rights-based approach may clash with other competing ethical and medical considerations. While issues of distributive justice have been debated over many years in health policy, it is a relatively recent consideration in terms of access to ARVs. And because these competing claims must be operationalized, South Africa's treatment guidelines are used to illustrate how significant ethical dilemmas arise. The chapter concludes by examining what a fair process in accessing ARVs might involve.

Rights-based Approaches to Access to Treatment and Health Care

With regard to achieving freedom from want, then, health is considered "a fundamental human right indispensable for the exercise of other human rights" (UN CESCR, General Comment 14, 2000). Article 12 of the International Covenant on Economic, Social and Cultural Rights (ICESCR) recognizes "the right of everyone to the enjoyment of the highest attainable standard of physical and mental health." In defining the scope of the "right to health," we can therefore divide this into two categories. One relates to "health care" as both curative and preventative. The other relates to the "underlying preconditions for health," including safe drinking water, adequate sanitation, adequate nutrition, health-related information, environmental health, and occupational health (Toebes 2001:174). The curative aspects of the right to health have been given special emphasis in recent years due to AIDS, resulting, as mentioned, in treatment being regarded as integral to the right to health. Activist pressure contributed to, and benefits from, efforts to clarify the relationship between treatment(s) more generally and the human right to health. Following Article 12 (2c) of the ICESCR, the availability of essential drugs is now regarded as an integral dimension of the right to health. The core content of the right to health therefore includes treatment, control of epidemics, as well as prevention.[1] In operationalizing the right to health, a useful starting point is to consider the following principles developed by Toebes (2001:177, 178):

- *Availability* of health services: the state must have a quantity of health services sufficient for the population as a whole.
- *Financial, geographic and cultural accessibility* of health services: financial accessibility requires that health services be affordable (and that there be an arrangement for the payment of health services for those who cannot afford the required care); geographic accessibility sets the requirement that they be within reach of everyone; and cultural accessibility, finally, necessitates that such services respect people's cultural traditions.
- *Quality* of health services: the available health services must be of adequate standard, which includes the requirement that the services be *appropriate* in the specific context.
- *Equality* in access to available health services: health services must be equally accessible to everyone, with due attention assigned to the position of vulnerable groups in society.

These aspects provide an important tool with which to provide leverage for, explore, and monitor access. A range of barriers to access is identified, namely, geographic, economic, cultural, and discriminatory ones in particular. Subsequent chapters look in more detail at these barriers. Without a deeper understanding of how the barriers are constituted, it remains unlikely that they will be undone simply by invoking human rights based principles and laws. Additional chapters will also seek to supplement the list of barriers to broaden this to include underemphasized dimensions of access. Notably, important additional dimensions include political accountability and governance of health institutions (Chapter 4); social and cultural attitudes within communities (chapters 5 and 6); and socioeconomic factors(Chapter 7); and selection critieria (Chapter 7). Elaborating on barriers to access suggests a need for increasing recognition of the interplay between human rights and broader developmental aspects. This is particularly the case, therefore, in understanding access in specific contexts (Chapter 3).

Farmer, for example, goes beyond the observation of barriers to more forcefully suggest that: "[N]o honest assessment of the current state of human rights can omit an analysis of structural violence"(Farmer 2005). That is, poverty and political violence and social inequality are products of acute race, gender, and class differences. These comprise structural determinants that disproportionately predispose the poor to vulnerability. As a consequence, this makes them more likely to suffer ill health. Farmer's work has contributed to broader efforts to link human rights to development problems and processes in what is often termed a *human rights-based approach to development*. At a basic level of understanding, international human rights norms and standards are increasingly being applied by NGOs and states and civil society organizations to problems historically considered the terrain of "development." Numerous authors indicate the benefits to both the human rights and development sectors from the overlap.[2] Jonsson (2005:60), for example, regards the approach as foregrounding human rights as both the objective and also as the process itself. Human rights standards can be used as benchmarks for desirable outcomes but they also represent conditions for the development process. The freedoms intrinsic to a liberal conception of human rights (civil and political rights) and related notions of nondiscrimination, accountability, and participation and equality are now being applied toward analyzing and tackling socioeconomic inequalities and social exclusion. This growing agenda has firmly (re)placed socioeconomic rights within development discourse and practice.

As mentioned previously, struggles around AIDS treatment have provided a tremendous force with which to return human rights to its more holistic interpretation in the Universal Declaration of Human Rights (UDHR). As many increasingly argue, how is it possible to talk about freedoms without also demanding freedom from want? Surely the lack of one impairs the optimal use of the other. If someone is starving or, dying from AIDS, it becomes very hard to see the value of voting or due process. On the other hand, socioeconomic rights are more likely to be met through political and civil means. But we should not underestimate how the struggle for material needs and structural violence conditions and impairs those "freedoms." Liberal democratic rights may not reduce social and economic inequality. On the contrary, they may even serve to legitimize inequality in the present neoliberal economic order (Evans 2002). Having said so, however, this appears to be dead-end analysis, devoid of the possibility of political struggles. In other words, following Jones and Stokke (2005), we can at least agree that these rights provide a more likely basis from which to seek to tackle inequality. Responses to the AIDS epidemic have historically recognized types of structural violence and discrimination leveled against people living with AIDS. As a result, the AIDS epidemic has been a catalyst for a human rights-based approach to health more generally. A rights-based approach, at its core, should be a political act in that duty-bearers are identified and their obligations demanded by claimants empowered by a rights discourse and practice. But all of this assumes, of course, that there is agreement in thinking on rights.

Thinking about Human Rights

Depicted as a necessary, even superior, set of normative values, human rights are far from neutral, nor uncontested. A useful starting point for conceptualizing human rights concerns separating out two essential characteristics at their core.[3] On the one hand, human rights derive from so-called natural law, literally deriving from a sense of a natural state of man *prior* to being shaped by social relations. A recurring theme, then, is how this natural condition provides a set of moral principles to govern our humanity: how we care for others and how they should treat us. We therefore have prior ethical entitlements or claims with which to, hopefully, safeguard this natural condition. Just as natural law provides the impetus in efforts to safeguard rights and freedoms, it is also a fundamental weakness in justifying rights. Undoubtedly, who decides them and, indeed, which ones are selected as fundamental rights can be contested. Similarly, how disagreements on rights are dealt with may change and be interpreted differently across different cultures also reflect the contested claims that human rights are simply universal. What features or moral attributes deemed to characterize a common humanity have been heavily disputed, rendering them, for many, akin to "a moral fiction." Some observers, such as Ignatief (2001), doubt whether genuine agreement can ever be reached on these core values of humanity. In many contexts, humanity is considered as realized not through a detached, consenting, rational individual, freed of the restrictions of authority but, instead perhaps, through communal or family relations. Others suggest that despite differences in "world views'" (or, '"ontological differences"), the emphasis on origins and foundations is considered to be misleading. Rather, a plurality of perspectives is regarded as highly compatible with a more fluid and poly-vocal base that reflects multicultural and religious diversity. Whilst therefore hard to pin down philosophically, and open to critique about their social fabrication, it is the sense of injustice felt when these values have been infringed that forms the core of human rights idealism and activism. While rights remain "a moral fiction," as Gready and Ensor (2005:3) suggest, however, "it can be a very empowering fiction, and has a profound political impact." And Ignatief also observes that while it may be impossible to agree on their foundations, it can be agreed that we need rights. It is this sense of protecting human agency and nurturing empowerment that continues to drive human rights onward. But how to do this and which rights are to be considered as a necessary common denominator to a core human rights project remains keenly contested.

The other dimension integral to its very core, then, concerns the translation of these ethical entitlements into social and political practice. In other words, lest we do harm to others, these natural laws cannot command unlimited freedoms because of the need to balance our own rights against the freedoms and rights of others. As a result of the need for creating social order, rights require organization beyond quasi-religious principles. This is the idea of a *social contract*, whereby rulers, states in particular, are bound by these human rights norms to govern by consent in return for placing certain boundaries on rights when these may be harmful to others. A profound historical shift takes place in liberal thought in the relationship between the individual and the state. Duties have become expected of rulers on the basis of legitimate claims of citizens who consent to restraints on freedoms for the common good. Rights have come to provide a mechanism of accountability against arbitrary and unjust state actions: rights therefore speak to the articulation and exercise of power.

The key point is that rights continue to evolve at the interface between natural law idealism and the pragmatism and problems of enforcement associated with the social contract and nation-building.[4] A critical proposal made here is that rights are therefore not only narrowly about laws and regulations alone but also firmly embedded in moral, social, and political processes that also comprise them. While there are fundamental differences between rights and democracy, for example, the political system of a country and political priorities will be particularly important for enabling human rights to be respected, protected, promoted, and fulfilled (Archibold 2003). Democracy is often contested and under strain from those either never included in a social contract, or, when the latter is not deemed to provide benefits (whether economic or political, or perhaps cultural). As a result, there is no guarantee that democracy will deliver or secure human rights. Human rights are indeterminate, however. Just as they can be co-opted and their language used by the more powerful, at times and under certain conditions, the excluded can also co-opt them. This is what can give rights their open-endedness and, hence, unpredictability. Liberal democracy does provide a necessary basis from which to seek the protection of rights but it is not a sufficient one, especially for socioeconomic rights, for their fulfillment (Jones and Stokke 2005).

Since the UDHR in 1948, far from being abstract principles, a considerable array of international human rights law has since been developed in the so-called Age of Rights. These human rights mechanisms give specific substance to rights in the form of standards that elaborate the rights and map out the corresponding obligations of states (Eide 2003). The UDHR reflects a specific historical juncture in the evolution of rights, namely, coming to terms with the horrors of the Second World War, the unfolding cold war, and a process wherein its drafting was prior to decolonization of most of the colonized world. It is therefore socially constructed and limited to a particular time and place. But for all these limitations, the UDHR was nonetheless the beginning of the modern era of human rights. It lays down the foundations for subsequent norms and standards. These have not remained static but have evolved in a more inclusive and holistic fashion to provide a fuller and still unfolding picture of humanity.

So, for example, contrary to the spirit of the UDHR that clearly considered political and civil rights and socioeconomic rights to be indivisible and interdependent (freedoms *and* freedom from want), these rights have been separated and treated very differently by the human rights community. In the Cold War era, an overtly liberal interpretation of rights was exaggerated by Western powers. One could easily argue that socioeconomic rights have unfairly and unnecessarily been demoted and downgraded, subordinate to civil and political rights (Jones and Stokke 2005). However, in more recent years, one notable exception has been AIDS activists who have used such standards of ethical entitlement to create a politics of the moral high ground to morally and publicly shame pharmaceutical companies over their profiteering through drug-pricing policies. The lack of access gave such moral force to campaigns precisely because this scientific technology existed, was available, but was out of reach for the global majority of people living with AIDS due to its cost. In seeking to prolong the life of people living with AIDS, campaigning for treatment has also been profound for reestablishing the interdependency and indivisibility of *all* human rights. Arguably, the restoration of human rights to how it was originally more holistically conceived has been greatly assisted by struggles to access socioeconomic rights, such as health and, within this, access to treatment (Jones and Stokke 2005).

As suggested, if human rights are to become and remain relevant they must also acknowledge other contexts. In a related fashion, therefore, while human rights purport to be about freedom, an obvious rejoinder is how different social and cultural systems may interpret freedom and liberal norms. Whereas certain practices may be valued for the dignity and communal belonging they bestow, in other quarters, they will be regarded as infringing basic liberal tenets. As mentioned earlier in this section, the philosophical foundations of human rights can be disputed and a liberal bias toward the rational and autonomous individual exposed and contested by interpretations focusing more on the collective or community level. Compatibility can be strived for and consent, tolerance, and adjudicating the harm of particular actions or practices are useful benchmarks for doing so. But such norms may clash with competing worldviews. In an interesting discussion of *virginity testing*, for example, Vincent makes the point that no matter how abhorrent the practice may be from a liberal perspective, it cannot necessarily be rejected if using the basis of the participant's lack of consent or because it is harmful to others (which she did not find). The overall point she makes, moreover, is that liberalism is not a neutral concept. Instead, it has an encoded voice of authority in placing its own values as those to be aspired to through creating "liberal selves." Alternatively, whilst this rights-based future is still to be attained and progressive citizens created, in the meantime, others may instead consider progress as representing a loss—whether in values, social stability, identity, or even life, in the case of AIDS (Vincent 2007). This gap between international human rights, national constitutional values, and culture and tradition tests the limits of rights-based approaches but is also an acknowledgment of their nonneutrality. Liberalism, paradoxically, can be more about asserting its own authority rather than freedoms. This leaves human rights open to a range of criticisms, not least that there is somehow an ideal citizen that we should all aspire—even be forced—to become renders rights as a necessary abstraction (Englund 2006). A more enlightened, less arrogant version of rights would at least seek to square respect for rights with respect for cultures insofar as the latter are compatible with human rights standards, such as nondiscrimination, for example. It could also seek to demonstrate that rights can be used to protect culture. However, whether we can avoid the encoded bias and authority inherent in human rights is less certain.

Arguably, then, although human rights exhibit a range of ambiguities, the historical evolution of ideas in rights reflects one of its great advantages: its fluid, evolutionary nature. This fluidity has seen the agenda of rights expand to incorporate issues of race, gender, class, and culture. Although these liberal norms collide at times with particular beliefs and values, they do provide a basis from which tolerance and nondiscrimination are more likely to achieve social, political, and cultural accommodation. And it is an accommodation that must remain flexible if rights are to be deemed legitimate. They also provide "a set of ground rules for society" (Archibold 2003:81). More radical conceptions of rights can also regard them as the basis for equality and social transformation (Jones and Stokke 2005). Not least, human rights have been particularly important in giving space and legitimacy to access to medication in the context of health care. Given the complex mediation of such universal ideals associated with human rights, however, it is perhaps inevitable that they, and associated concepts like democracy, are conditioned by very different processes and geographic contexts. Ironically, as a rights-based approach to the epidemic and to development becomes more prominent, they are also receiving greater scrutiny.

For some critics, like Englund (2006), for example, there is an apparent inability to acknowledge the messiness of situating abstract concepts like human rights within specific contexts. The result is that human rights discourse and practitioners can themselves serve to depoliticize the exercise of power. This is because "human rights," for example, are demarcated by proponents and antagonists alike, who prefer to keep them abstract in order to enable promotion of their own interests. Understanding this process, whereby transformatory concepts are tamed and hijacked is impossible without, for Englund, some historical understanding of state elite behavior. In his country case study, Malawi, for example, the continuity between colonial and postcolonial social systems and values is particularly significant. Even human rights activists fall to the temptation to mimic elite behavior that is historically engrained. In an ethnographic study, he demonstrates some of the different arenas within which there is a deliberate attempt to keep these concepts abstract. He notes, for example, the specific role played by poor translation of human rights instruments into local dialects and the ineffectiveness of the human rights and democracy workshops observed and failures of legal aid. These are kept abstract, he claims, because they lend themselves to maintaining social hierarchy. The broader point that Englund makes is that the critique that concepts like human rights and democracy should bring with them is not allowed in the rules of the game as defined by elites and intermediaries. Ordinary people are not allowed to participate in defining these terms. Participants therefore remain "prisoners of freedom" because human rights and freedom are the preoccupation of the privileged few and a basis for creating exclusions and inclusions in power.

Similarly, and more specifically in terms of rights-based approaches to ARV treatment, Høg (2006) observes that despite the prevalence of a rights-based policy framework in Mozambique, human rights in this arena more broadly reflect a "silence on rights." Rights are poorly disseminated, understood, and translated into local language due to a number of cultural, social, and political reasons. Politically, here as in other countries, a state is seen to subscribe to a rights-based agenda but whilst paradoxically attempting to exert its own bureaucratic and sovereign control. Not least, for civil society, rather than rights-based claims, there is instead a social system premised upon a particular social hierarchy that must be navigated with skill and diplomacy. Political actors must therefore be courted in an appropriate cultural way, "recognising and addressing the 'right' persons and high-level politicians with the most polite and correct wording and transactional rituals" (p. 54). As reflected in their limited use for advocacy and public discussion, for Høg, this "silence of rights" explains their weak performance power. The apparent disjuncture between rights and popular perceptions of them is noticeable in a range of country contexts. It is also looked at in the next chapter specifically addressing Hammanskraal-Temba.

The challenges posed to human rights approaches as discussed in the Introduction, and chapters 1 and 2 are considerable. The chapters that follow all suggest the specific social, political, geographic, and cultural contexts that must therefore be openly acknowledged rather than denied. The conclusion will also respond in terms of whether a different reality is possible for human rights.

To talk, though, of "universal access" to medication inevitably shows up the divergences between the universal ideals of concepts like human rights, and ethical, pragmatic, and political contexts of policy execution.

Universal Access

The most influential global policy approach to date concerning access to AIDS medication was the World Health Organization's "3 by 5" campaign. This aimed to provide access to AIDS medication to 3 million people by 2005. WHO's objective was to expand access, understood as universal access *"for everyone who requires it according to medical criteria."*[5] But the partial coverage, both globally and within and between provinces in countries like South Africa, inevitably qualifies what "universal access" means in substantive terms. In other words, certain groups and areas are less likely to get access than others. It was shown in the previous chapter that South Africa's Constitutional Court deemed the government to be unreasonably blocking access to the AIDS drug, Nevirapine. Expectant mothers and their newborn babies were not allowed to make use of the drug because access was restricted. "Access," in this sense, can therefore be understood as "able to get, have, or use something." "To have access" means that *government must facilitate access or create an enabling environment for everyone to access a service.*[6] In addition to health, a number of other socioeconomic rights (land, housing, food and water, and social security) in the South African

Constitution are often phrased in terms of "to have access to" the right in question.[7] It alludes to enabling a process or environment, a "qualified right," rather than a direct right to the service or product in question. In the Nevirapine case, the court clearly felt that the ability to get, have, or use treatment was denied by government's restrictions on it. Removing unnecessary restrictions is one important aspect of access. But ensuring that people are actually able to access the good, service, or information in question is another.

WHO does acknowledge this in referring to the need for "protecting and serving vulnerable groups in prevention and treatment programs." In fact, WHO states in one of the eleven guiding principles of the "3 by 5" initiative that "the initiative will make special efforts to ensure access to antiretroviral therapy for people who risk exclusion because of economic, social, geographical or other barriers." Again, while acknowledging that barriers to access occur, this is not firmed up in the initiative. The latter therefore did not specify how equity would be achieved or unfairness minimized. WHO documents do refer to better use of key "entry points" such as TB patients who may be coinfected with AIDS and therefore require treatment but are already within the medical system. But the documents do not detail means of prioritizing social criteria for selection of patients (WHO 2003a). A discussion paper prepared for a follow-up meeting on the implementation of the United Nations 2001 Declaration of Commitment on HIV/AIDS does, however, mention structural factors such as lack of skilled health-care workers and "the barriers to access presented by cost-recovery mechanisms [in other words, the charging of fees for patients to access services]."[8]

Barriers to access are also invoked in some detail in rights-specific documents. For example, the "International Guidelines on HIV/AIDS and Human Rights," in the commentary on revised guideline number six states that "universal access requires that these goods, services and information [that is, concerning prevention, care and treatment] not only be available, acceptable and of good quality but also within physical reach and affordable for all."[9] It also identifies the need for positive measures "to address factors that hinder equal access," such as poverty, migration, rural location, and "discrimination of various kinds." Although not elaborated upon, in these documents, the identification of some barriers raises important issues concerning access to ARVs.[10] So, if we take a holistic view of access, we can flag those elements needed to better reflect issues in access. In particular, I would propose adding:

- First, *political accessibility*, in terms of the accountability of the process.
- Second, *institutional accessibility*, particularly in terms of both workplace and community and institution relations for understanding quality of the service.

- Third, in addition to socioeconomic barriers, the *social acceptability* of the service in question is also important.
- Finally, culture appropriateness is mentioned, but what does that actually entail for cultural accessibility of services?

Some observers therefore suggest that the role originally envisaged for human rights in ARV policy has in fact been disappointing. Rights appear to be quite marginalized in the treatment era (Gruskin et al 2007). I would agree with these authors that we are far from creating a genuine rights-based approach to treatment policy and implementation. The benefits of such an approach have not been permitted to flourish. In part, this is perhaps been due to a failure to contextualize rights within the complex processes and structures encountered in societies. Rather than acknowledging this complexity, there is instead a growing tendency to throw the rights-baby out with the bathwater and simply to move on to yet another paradigm. What is suggested here instead is the need to negotiate the messiness when rights are placed in a specific context. As mentioned above, additional barriers discussed here include political, social, and cultural acceptability in addition to socioeconomic barriers. But other barriers human rights encounter also concern competing ethical and medical claims in setting criteria for selection for treatment. As expressed by both donors and civil society alike, the criteria used to determine "who" will receive it and on what criteria basis are not clear or unambiguous.[11]

As Simple as "First Come, First Served"?: Considerations and Criteria in Selection

Clinical criteria for accessing ARVs, such as CD4 counts and viral load tests, are well established. A much more vague area concerns in what circumstances nonclinical factors should also be considered in defining eligibility for access to ARVs. Rationing, for example, might be required for all those clinically eligible for ARVs but demand is too high in relation to supply of the drugs in high prevalence countries. There is the danger that those patients—like those mentioned in the introduction in Zambia—who are already better placed in society might maximize their access to ARVs, while those more vulnerable may not be able to.[12] The "first come, first served" principal appears intrinsically fair. However, if we accept that there is a more general tendency of governance decision-making and policy to prejudice the poorer and more vulnerable in society, then this qualifies how fair it can be. More specifically, health interventions "seldom reach the poor" and HIV/AIDS focuses attention on the "skewed distribution of basic health services within and between countries."[13] The built-in structural bias against the poor, while a major consideration in access, is but one of many. The Chairman of the Commission on HIV and Governance in

Africa, K. Y. Amoako, has raised the specter of what he called "antiretroviral anarchy" across the continent. This anarchy would not only be premised upon the most privileged receiving access. In addition, diversion to black market sales and irrational prescription and growing drug resistance would all contribute.[14] Whether treatment programs will reinforce social inequalities, challenge them, or, at the very least, be considered "fair" and acceptable places great stock in the criteria created and how they are created.

According to the review by Jones (2005b), it would therefore appear important to explore these criteria. Table 2.1 provides a synthesis of a range of criteria. It shows how criteria may encompass "first come, first served" principles and many other considerations. A patient's occupation (such as state employees getting preference, i.e., health care workers, teachers, army, police, and civil servants) may be a significant claim. Certainly, where the patient is located and the geography of access (usually geographically defined residence and/or in building upon existing capacity, catering mainly to urban areas) will also have a bearing on access. Other factors include whether to prioritize expectant mothers in building upon prevention of mother-to-child transmission programs. For others, children will be a priority. There may also be good medical reasons to target those already receiving TB treatment or those with a better likelihood of a positive medical outcome, and so on.

The issue of barriers to access is also particularly significant in a context of continuing and widespread stigma and discrimination associated with the epidemic. It should therefore be important to ask what may happen when adjudicating the access to ARVs of stigmatized social groups such as sex workers; injecting drug users, and men having sex with men, orphans, alcoholics, or others with social problems. Whether they will be judged as "deserving" or "undeserving" is a particular concern. Table 2.1 includes criteria to address "ethical/rights-based" issues. A fundamental point to be made is that, on the contrary, rights-based principles are not necessarily the same as other criteria. A brief comment is provided alongside each criterion in the table.

Clearly, then, flagging-up some issues in criteria setting serves to illustrate some of the difficulties in prioritizing between these different criteria. It is particularly important to seek to ask questions about the social, cultural, and political acceptability involved in defining criteria and monitoring programs. Above all, to what extent is information provided deemed acceptable? The quality and consistency of information would also go a long way in removing unacceptable dimensions of political, social, and cultural practices. These, of course, are not criteria per se but they should certainly be used, first, to discuss criteria setting, and, second, monitor programs. As this process is heavily value-laden and immensely complicated suggests the need for adjudication. As suggested, this is a relatively recent issue receiving attention in the context of ARVs. The following sections will also refer to Table 2.1. Treatment guidelines constitute

Table 2.1 Ethical and rights-based criteria in access to ARVs

Criteria	*Comment*
Clinical (As defined by WHO regarding CD4 count etc., and adapted for low-resource settings)	Debate concerning biomedical criteria, with evidence of a need for flexibility in criteria setting in low-resource settings.
Efficiency Likelihood of adherence Prioritizing those already tested versus those not yet tested Expectant mothers/plus those receiving treatment through prevention of MTCT programs And/or those already receiving TB Treatment	Here it could be argued that it is more efficient to target those who already know status, and children and partners of pregnant women. But does this penalize nonpregnant women?
Economic	Those who can make a financial contribution to subsidized medication—but what about the poorest of the poor?
Social/Geographic "First come, first served" Women's access through MTCT prevention programs Time-keeping of patient appointments Eligibility through local residency Degree of disclosure Likelihood of adherence PLWA number of dependents Community selection committees	Raises issues of whether there is bias toward better educated/informed, urban, often men? Will there be specific measures to overcome barriers to access, e.g., travel, female targeting, finances, awareness raising, particularly through "treatment literacy"? Women's access might then outstrip men's access, as appears to be the case in sub-Saharan Africa Time-keeping and some disclosure may heighten efficiency, and adherence may be the key consideration Eligibility through geography may be exclusionary, especially in transitory populations Are those less likely to adhere being denied access? Community participation in selection committees appears transparent but may encourage bias/corruption
Rights-based Criteria should reflect: Non-discrimination Concern for vulernable social groups Political acceptability Social Acceptability Cultural Acceptability Information acceptability *Ethical claims* Post-exposure prophylaxis for health care workers, and women and children exposed through rape or sexual abuse Those too sick to travel to hospital/clinic Poorest of the poor Those whose drugs trials end	Groups such as men who have sex with men, sex workers, orphans, migrant workers and refugees–special targeting because they are marginalized and may be considered "undeserving" by society Bed-ridden at home also excluded But is this compatible with determining a more efficient outcome, adherence?
Administrative/political State employees getting preference	Due to burden upon states of cost of absenteeism/death

the initial operationalization of such criteria for patients seeking access to treatment. They are therefore significant in enabling or preventing access.

Treatment Guidelines and the Ethical and Clinical Dimensions Surrounding Access

A critical caveat to "macro" debates concerning ARV provision concerns the internal political process of creating a national treatment plan and national AIDS structures, such as AIDS councils, within individual countries. One fundamental consideration is how willing—and able—national governments are to fulfill their obligations to provide treatment in a manner compatible with equity principles of "macro" guidelines.[15] The extent to which national treatment plans reflect public debate, transparent decision-making processes, access to information, and strong multi-sectoral cooperation and committed leadership are critical in a "fair process" in ARV access.[16] With few exceptions,[17] it is rather surprising, then, that there is a paucity of analysis in drawing these "macro" guidelines down into specific national contexts.

An initial starting point is to consider and reflect upon the process involved in creating selection criteria in South Africa. In 2004, for example, the former head of the Department of Health's Directorate of STI and HIV/AIDS, Dr. Simelela, gave a seminar presentation of the, then, newly launched operational plan. After the presentation, I posed a question: "Was the government considering the benefits of using social and equity based criteria as a proactive measure to create more equitable access to ARVs?" and "were these considerations in the implementation of the plan?" In reply, Simelela stated that such criteria had been considered by a panel of constitutional and legal experts prior to the final drafting of treatment guidelines.[18] Apparently, the fear of additional litigation, based on specific rights and equality and nondiscrimination clauses in particular, appeared to be the spur for government's scrutiny of social criteria. And, these social criteria, she replied, were deemed unconstitutional because they might impair constitutional values. But, contrary to WHO, as will be shown (see "South Africa's Operational Plan"), the South Africa criteria *are* nonetheless inherently related to the predicted likelihood of adherence (and hence the medical efficiency criteria in Table 2.1), itself a *de facto* criteria.

Regarding predictions of adherence in influencing patient selection, for example, WHO policy can be found in two documents: a set of ethical guidelines entitled, "Guidance on ethics and equitable access to HIV treatment and care" and a set of clinical guidelines called, "Scaling up antiretroviral therapy in resource-limited settings: Treatment guidelines for a public health approach–2003 revision." WHO's ethical guidelines specifically condemn the practice of denying ARVs to patients believed to be at high risk of nonadherence. They recommend that patients facing adherence barriers be provided with the special assistance they need to overcome these obstacles. WHO's recommendations stand in sharp contrast to South Africa's own ARV policy, which is embodied in the government's "National antiretroviral treatment guidelines" (the "ARV guidelines") and in the more general "Operational plan for comprehensive HIV and AIDS care, management and treatment for South Africa" (the "HIV/AIDS care plan").

Despite the contrary intentions of at least some members of its drafting committee, the South Africa ARV guidelines appear to suffer from ambiguity. They could be read as permitting, or even encouraging, the use of predicted nonadherence to exclude patients from ARV. One of the drafters, Dr. Francois Venter,[19] head of the Clinicians Society of Southern Africa, suggests that the ARV guidelines were never intended for health care providers to either advocate or permit the exclusion of patients based on predictions of nonadherence. Both Venter and the other drafters made clear that adherence is basically unpredictable. By his account, the drafters emphasized potential barriers to adherence only because they hoped to get nurses and patients thinking about these barriers and to induce patients to accept responsibility for adhering. However, Dr. Venter does agree that the guidelines can be used to exclude patients from treatment because health care providers may be overcautious and prone to interpreting the guidelines "biblically." Furthermore, the guidelines may also be used as a convenient mechanism to reduce strain on inadequate resources. Finally, according to Venter, many health care providers have received insufficient training on them. The question that still remains, however, is whether these guidelines are serving to exclude.

Health care providers may feel that the guidelines mandate both support groups and frequent appointments for each and every patient. The guidelines are regarded as "a local refinement" of WHO recommendations. That is, they differ from those recommendations only in that the guidelines recognize that South Africa's comparatively greater resources permits it to do things—like more comprehensive monitoring of viral loads—that other countries cannot do.[20] For Venter, the most important obstacles to universal access to ARV are operational, not clinical. Whatever the intentions of its drafters, South Africa's "National antiretroviral treatment guidelines" do not appear to take a clear stand against the denial of ARV based on predictions of nonadherence. At best, the ARV guidelines contradict themselves when addressing the matter. At worst, they may leave health care providers with the impression that ARV should in fact be denied to patients who are perceived unlikely to adhere to the treatment program.

In South Africa, treatment criteria are stated according to the "National antiretroviral treatment guidelines,"[21] which, more recently, in 2008, have been revised in the "Guidelines for the management of HIV & AIDS in health facilities."[22] The two main areas of criteria are as follows (with significant revisions in 2008 in italics):

First is the commonly used medical or clinical criteria:

- CD4 count < 200 cells/mm3 (*revised to 250 cells/mm3*) irrespective of WHO stage; or
- WHO stage 4 disease irrespective of CD4 count.

Second is a range of additional factors termed "psychosocial":

- Demonstrated reliability, i.e., has attended three or more scheduled visits to an HIV clinic
- No active alcohol or other substance abuse
- No untreated active depression
- Disclosure: it is strongly recommended that clients have disclosed their HIV status to at least one friend or family member OR have joined a support group.
- *If possible the patient should identify a treatment supporter who should also receive information and be educated on HAART.*
- Insight: Clients need to have accepted their HIV positive status, and have insight into the consequences of HIV infection and the role of ARV treatment before commencing ARV therapy (including nonadherence).
- Able to attend the antiretroviral center on a regular basis (transport may need to be arranged for patients in rural areas or for those remote from the treatment site) or have access to services able to maintain the treatment chain.

The psychosocial criteria appear to be based upon efforts to enhance efficacy and adherence of the treatment, that is, medical efficacy. Whilst, of course, efficacy and adherence are important objectives, it should be noted that there are not the same as equity criteria. The latter can be based upon human rights and ethical considerations concerning the most vulnerable—the poorest—which may be contrary to efficiency arguments. In other country contexts reflecting a high prevalence of HIV and scarcity of resources, other criteria may be used, for example, giving state employees preferential treatment. Although the psychosocial criteria are stated as factors not to be used to exclude patients, whether they are or are not used to exclude perhaps requires close scrutiny. Furthermore, regarding patient selection, it is stated that "the final decision to treat will be taken by the multidisciplinary team at the ARV centre, who will initiate treatment." This raises additional issues of who the team is and how they reach decisions for accepting or rejecting patients for treatment.

This, and the absence of equity considerations, does suggest the need to monitor who is or is not receiving treatment in terms of disaggregated information based upon gender, age, perhaps socioeconomic circumstances, and location, for example, where the treatment is provided (clinic or hospital, for example) against prevalence figures. These facets involved in monitoring equity have featured as important demands made by the Joint Civil Society Monitoring Forum to government.[23] However, data is still hard to come by. There is therefore also a need to assess the barriers encountered by people living with AIDS in qualitative terms (Chapters 3 through 7). In this way, specific measures to enhance equity may be identified and promoted. But Section 1 of the guidelines, for example, which addresses ARV for adult patients, is plagued by mixed messages. The authors do note, within a set of parentheses, that the psycho-social considerations are "not exclusion criteria." However, this attempt at clarification is contradicted by other more prominent messages contained in the text.

First, the psychosocial considerations could hardly constitute "patient selection criteria" if they were not at least sometimes meant to have bearing upon whether a patient is selected for treatment. Second, the guidelines tell health care providers that "the multi-disciplinary team [responsible for deciding whether to initiate ARV] should meet" before a patient's second visit in order to "assess patient readiness." The team "should take all available information into account" when making this assessment. Furthermore, "patients who do not meet the treatment readiness criteria should be referred back to their local clinic with a detailed letter" articulating the "reason for deferment of ARV." These aspects of the text create ample space for an interpretation permitting the exclusion of patients whose psycho-social considerations indicate barriers to adherence. Section 2 suffers from even more serious problems. As in section 1, the authors parenthetically note that the psycho-social considerations are, again, "not exclusion criteria."[24] However, the psycho-social considerations are nonetheless placed under the heading, "Selection of patients for antiretroviral therapy" and are identified as "criteria for commencing ARV in children." Even more worrying are the authors' claims that "children being considered for ARV will need to meet *both* medical and psycho-social criteria before starting therapy" (emphasis added), that the psycho-social considerations "are extremely important for the success of the programme . . . and need to be adhered to," and that "the principle" for health care providers to keep in mind "is that adherence must be at least probable." While section 1 leaves room for the exclusion of patients failing to meet the psycho-social criteria, section 2 all but mandates such exclusions.

In the revised guidelines, Mr. T. D. Mseleku, director-general of the Department of Health, states that adherence should receive even greater attention (2008:5): "Adherence to HAART is of paramount importance to reaping the long-term benefits and avoiding development of resistance. Maximum adherence requires community mobilization with patients supported by health care providers, family and the community to participate and fully understand the benefit and limitations of HAART. The National public health programme boasts one of the highest treatment retention rates in the world. In order to optimise these outcomes and reduce the risks of drug toxicity and resistance, it is imperative that this remarkable achievement is sustained."

In drawing attention to the emphasis given to adherence, the purpose, again, is in no way to deny the obvious benefits of adhering. Rather, it is to suggest whether this is asking an awful lot of patients to access ARVs. Not least, a paradigm of "community mobilization" and "participation" implies that a degree of disclosure is apparently preferred. This should therefore raise the question of what burdens these criteria—if exercised literally—may have on people living with AIDS. Not least, how might they be having the effect of filtering out patients who encounter particularly difficult levels of social difficulties? We could also add to these, the role of judgments based on social attitudes. It is not uncommon to hear from people living with AIDS, such as one at his local clinic in Tzaneen, in Limpopo Province, of cases whereby staff "refuse" patients treatment if they do not, for example, come with a "treatment buddy." Some of these exclusions related to "psycho-social criteria" are pursued in Chapter 7 in the context of Hammanskraal-Temba.[25]

The ARV guidelines approach WHO policy most closely in section 3, which addresses "antiretroviral treatment adherence." Here, the authors make known their belief that "it is not possible for health care providers to reliably predict which individuals will ultimately be adherent to their treatment plan." However, the authors seem more worried about unreliable predictions of adherence than about those of nonadherence. Health care providers are told that "it is essential to provide all patients with a comprehensive plan to support adherence." that "there is evidence that there is less adherence as time progresses," and that monitoring and ongoing support of adherence is essential." Each of these statements aims to disabuse health care providers of the notion that they may ever rely upon a prediction of adherence by trusting a patient to adhere in the absence of outside monitoring and support. Nowhere in section 3 do the guidelines make clear that health care providers may not rely upon a prediction of nonadherence by refusing to initiate ARV.

South Africa's Operational Plan for Comprehensive HIV and AIDS Care, Management, and Treatment

Unlike the ARV guidelines, the HIV/AIDS care plan suffers little from ambiguity. Unfortunately, however, the very clear message communicated by the care plan is that ARV should be denied to patients who appear unlikely to adhere. This message is contained in the care plan's provisions on ARV initiation for both adults and children:

> The indication for antiretroviral treatment is based on clinical assessment and CD4 count. These important factors determine whether therapy should be started, or if it can be delayed. The lower the CD4 count, the higher the risk of AIDS and the more urgent the need for treatment. However, the risk of developing AIDS must be weighed against the risks of toxicity and development of resistance. Guidelines for eligibility criteria provide reference . . . (see Table 1.1) but must be considered along with individual patient readiness for starting treatment. Patients must be prepared to make a lifelong commitment to taking ARVs, which may require not only education to gain understanding of potential side-effects and importance of adherence, but also psychosocial support to overcome fears. Well-informed and engaged patients are the most successful with adherence to therapy. *The decision to initiate therapy must therefore be based not only on meeting the criteria and being ready to start, but also on being committed to adhering to treatment over the long term* (emphasis added).[26]
>
> Just as with adults, the decision to start treatment in children must take into account patient readiness along with the clinical and CD4 eligibility criteria. In the case of infants and children, "patient readiness" refers to readiness of the responsible person who will be administering the ARV drugs. It is mandatory that at least one responsible person be present who is capable of ensuring adherence to the child's ARV schedule. Other factors that may be considered by the health care team to determine treatment readiness, include: primary health clinic attendance record, immunization record, and previous history of medication compliance (anti-TB, nutritional supplementation). Clinical and CD4 eligibility criteria for starting therapy are listed in Table 1.4.

Tables 1.1 and 1.4 referenced in the text quoted above confirm that the HIV/AIDS care plan incorporates predictions of adherence into its criteria for initiation of ARV:

1.1 Criteria for ARV Initiation in Adults and Adolescentsing pregnant women

- CD4 < 200 cells/ mm3 and symptomatic, irrespective of stage, *or*
- WHO stage IV AIDS defining illness, irrespective of CD4 count, *and*
- Patient prepared and ready to take ARVs adherently

. . .

1.4 Criteria for ARV Initiation in Children < 6 Years Old

- CD4 < 15% and symptomatic, *or*
- WHO Paediatric Stage III AIDS defining illness, irrespective of CD4 %, *and*
- At least one responsible person capable of administering child's medication

Presumably, it is correct to assume that the drafters of South Africa's ARV guidelines never intended for health care providers to interpret the guidelines as authorizing the denial of ARV to patients believed unlikely to adhere to the treatment program. However, this interpretation is, at the very least, permitted by the actual text of the guidelines and even mandated by the government's HIV/AIDS care plan. It should come as no surprise if some public health care providers are under the impression that the South African government wishes for them to withhold ARV from patients facing serious adherence issues. A faithful reading of state policy could hardly have led them to any other conclusion.

Above all, in key WHO and UNAIDS and South African policy documents, there also appears to be something of a paradox of identification of—largely rhetorical, it must be said—statements about barriers to access but without any targeted measures necessary to alleviate them. Perhaps these have been subsumed in the policy urgency of accelerating technical delivery. The overall emphasis upon treatment readiness and adherence has important implications in terms of addressing social factors. But the ethical slippage apparent, namely, that they remain subordinate to medical efficacy, appears to (re)impose a dominant biomedical model upon treatment. What consequences this has for people living with AIDS is examined in the final chapter. But in the meantime, are there any working examples which have incorporated debate on social and ethical considerations and, if so, how do they negotiate such dilemmas?

Notable Exceptions in Consideration of Ethical Claims

In Khayelitsha, outside Cape Town, Medecin Sans Frontieres (MSF), for example, have certain medical, social, and adherence criteria required for patients to commence ARV treatment. First, patients need to be on time for four appointments. Second, if necessary, they should undergo TB treatment prior to receiving ARVs. Third, with the overall goal stated as to achieve better outcomes through adherence to ARVs, this involves assessment of eligibility for commencing ARVs, including: a home visit to verify geographic eligibility and disclosure to at least one confident (over eighteen years of age, most likely a family member) who will act as a "treatment assistant." There is also emphasis placed upon commitment to long-term therapy and safe sex practices. Other factors may also be included such as the number of dependents and health status—with the very sick getting priority; income level (targeting the very poor as opposed to those being able to afford treatment); and, as stated, willingness to disclose; and perhaps prioritization if the patient has experience of political activism. These issues pose considerable dilemmas for MSF staff, and patients. Jumping queues, for example, even when medically justified, does mean that those still waiting may risk deterioration in their own health the longer they have to wait. Similarly, disclosing also presents considerable trauma for some patients, perhaps placing them at risk of physical violence or social exclusion. Macklin concurs that disclosure to family may be reasonable. But she regards additional criteria, such as home visits and membership of a support group, as violating the "ethical principle that requires choosing 'the least restrictive alternative' when it comes to limitations on an individual's freedom or privacy" (p. 317). The trade-off between adherence and confidentiality is evident. But perhaps Macklin underestimates the burden of trauma in disclosing, and, indeed the difficulties more generally involved in the process to enroll on treatment programs. Political activism might previously have been a prominent consideration in selection consideration but where does this leave others with similarly strong claims of their social "use" (public sector employees for example, see Table 2.1) or, those deemed less or, not, "useful." Dilemmas abound.

It is therefore particularly useful to consider the very thoughtful, open, and honest account of these terrible dilemmas as acknowledged by MSF's Khayelitsha program. Fox and Goemaere (2006:305) say, "In principle, fulfilment of *all* medical, social, and adherence criteria is required for beginning ARV treatment." However, they also suggest, rather confusingly, that actual practice dictates otherwise. The inclination of MSF staff is toward admitting patients even if they do not meet certain criteria—for example, if patients might not be able to stick to condom use and safe sex because they would like to have a baby. Fortunately, some of these dilemmas have become less of an issue because certain criteria, such as the geographic one, have been abandoned as treatment becomes increasingly accessible across South Africa. But Macklin therefore raises an interesting point in asking, if all are admitted, why then do MSF persist with a set of social and adherence criteria; why not just call it "first come, first served"? (Macklin, 2006). In other words, it appears that MSF is reluctant to simply call it "first come first served." This is because they continue to accept that some awareness of competing criteria is still required to inform selection.

Indeed, their valuable experience from Khayelitsha is merely a microcosm, they claim, of the problems encountered nationwide in the process of "scaling-up." These selection problems will persist and even become amplified, leaving them to suggest the following: "Expanding AIDS treatment on a national scale is an intricate public health challenge. A distributive ethics, oriented to benefit the greatest number of persons in all regions, communities, economic, social, and cultural groups in the country will have to prevail over an individual ethic that gives precedence to the well-being of each patient in a one-on-one relationship with health care professionals. It is likely to be accompanied by areas of tension between them" (Fox and Goemaere 2006: 311).

Clearly, there are competing ethical claims. Macklin, in some of her other work, therefore attaches great significance to consideration of these, even when not always conducive to equity, or medical efficacy (Macklin 2004). Some of the competing principles Macklin proposes are listed below and to some extent complement those in Table 2.1, for example:

- *Utility maximization* foregrounds greater efficiency—economic, social, or, medical—such as in treating those already tested and/or prioritizing those regarded as having the best chances of benefiting medically, or maximizing the social good. More controversial is the utilitarian principle that could be applied to groups considered to be the most productive and whose prioritization could maximize the "societal good." This could be health care workers, civil servants, activists, or, mothers, amongst others, depending on interpretation of social utility.
- Then there is the *egalitarian* principle of equity that seeks to maximize health equity. Again, as Macklin points out, it is less clear what it is that should be equalized: resources for health, health status, or access to health care? A simple observation would be to note that if equal resources were to be allocated for people living with AIDS, this would be inequitable for those people living with AIDS facing additional health needs, such as meningococcal meningitis, or TB and malaria.
- Whilst the fundamental requirement for equity is that all groups and persons have equal access to ARVs, determining who is "worst off," or least advantaged, the so-called *Maximin* principle is also problematic. This might apply to the sickest (those bedridden, at home, and unable to get to the clinic, for example) but this then is in conflict with both utility—i.e. those considered most suitable—and egalitarian principles.
- Then there is the *justice as reciprocity or compensation* principle. Here, there might be a call for providing something for the contributions people have made, such as individuals involved in clinical trials, or, those who suffered as a result of unsterile medical practices, negligence, and so on. In terms of "justice as reciprocity," there is the possibility that it recreates

notions of the "deserving" and "undeserving" infected and hence reinscribes stigmatizing attitudes mentioned earlier.

These difficult moral, ethical, and policy dilemmas therefore confirm Macklin's view "that there is no one right solution to this quandary" (Macklin 2006:320). In this, her involvement in WHO deliberation on treatment guidelines has been timely and influential.

WHO's ethical guidelines on adherence and ARV initiation are stated clearly and prominently in the title of section 4.4: "Presumed adherence should not be a criterion for prioritizing patients'" WHO (2004a). Reflecting Macklin's input, this position is supported with two arguments, one epistemic and one egalitarian in nature. WHO first claims that "predictions of nonadherence are unreliable" and that the practice of "denying [patients] access to ARV" based on such predictions is therefore "ethically problematic because denials based on unreliable predictions amount to unfair discrimination." WHO then buttresses this claim with an assertion that even if "future adherence could be accurately determined, the exclusion of patients with predicted problems of adherence would be questionable because" such exclusions "would exacerbate existing inequities." Factors that may contribute to nonadherence include "poverty, homelessness, lack of family support, and substance use and dependence." These factors are found disproportionately among those in the greatest need of help from society. A norm in favor of "fairness to the least well-off would require special measures in order to improve adherence among" such patients, not a policy "excluding them from ARV." This conclusion is backed up elsewhere in the ethical guidelines. The guidelines' fifth and sixth recommendations call on countries "to identity vulnerable, marginalized, or other potentially underserved populations" and to "consider the need for special policies and outreach programmes to prioritize these groups and to overcome barriers to their accessing care." The guidelines also include a section called, "Special efforts are required to ensure access to ARV for the poor," in which poverty is defined "in the broadest sense, beyond income poverty and including social and political exclusion."

WHO's egalitarian argument, if applied to an ARV program facing resource constraints, implies that the policy goal of minimizing aggregate HIV-related morbidity and mortality should at least sometimes yield to concerns of equity. A patient requiring "special measures" to overcome adherence barriers also requires a special investment of resources in order to attain an estimated probability of adherence equal to those who do not require special efforts. For a policymaker concerned solely with aggregate health outcomes, such a patient would represent a low-yield investment. WHO's ideal policymaker must thus sometimes be willing to compromise public health goals out of fidelity to egalitarian principles. It recognizes that "spending resources on nonadherent patients can reduce the benefit, in terms of health outcomes, produced by an ARV programme." More importantly, it concedes that the policy goals of "maximizing overall benefits and giving everyone a fair chance . . . are sometimes at odds" and declares that "an ARV programme may not invoke the justification of 'utility' to follow policies which, considered as a whole, deprive . . . vulnerable groups of a fair opportunity to get treatment and care for HIV."

Though less explicit than the ethical guidelines, the clinical guidelines could not reasonably be construed to permit denials of ARV based on anticipated nonadherence. Early in the guidelines, WHO identifies three "key tenets" that should underpin the management of public ARV program (WHO 2004b). The first of these tenets is that ARV program should be scaled-up "with a view to universal access, i.e. [that] all persons requiring treatment as indicated by medical criteria should have access to it." The guidelines never waver from this call for universal access. Adherence is not even mentioned in section three of the guidelines: "When to start ARV therapy in adults and adolescents." Instead, "anticipated patient adherence" is listed as a factor to be considered only "in the selection of ARV regimens."[27] Like the ethical guidelines, the clinical guidelines also suggest special measures, not exclusion, for patients facing adherence barriers. For example, the guidelines make clear that "[t]he clinical and immunological criteria for initiating [ARV in] substance-dependent patients do not differ from those in the general recommendations." "[I]njecting drug users who are eligible for ARV should therefore be guaranteed access to this life-saving therapy." WHO recommends that "special considerations" be made to deal with "lifestyle instability that challenges drug adherence" among this population, suggesting the resource-intensive option of "directly observed therapy" that "integrate[s] care of drug dependence (including drug substitution therapy) and HIV." Nowhere in the clinical guidelines does the WHO so much as imply that a prospectively nonadherence patient should ever be denied treatment. This stands somewhat in contrast to the South African guideline mentioned earlier. But the intention has been to problematize access in this chapter and, above all, to point to the huge significance attached to creating a "fair process" surrounding access to ARVs.

Fair Process and Participation

WHO (2002a, 2002b) and UNAIDS' (1996) guidelines are undoubtedly an important guide for AIDS policy responses and in laying out appropriate national institutional and legislative frameworks. A considerable challenge—following ongoing processes surrounding criteria setting and creating institutional frameworks—is, then, how to ensure that service delivery at the local scale is in accordance with the rights-based principles. Lack of resources, strained infrastructure and, above all, according to Fox and Goemaere, limited human resources in the form of doctors and nurses, pose huge barriers to expanding access (Fox and Goemaere (2006). These important issues notwithstanding, a rights-based perspective gives emphasis to the steps and commitments that governments can take to attain the progressive realization of the right to health. In other words, how ARV programs maximize equity and minimize unfairness and barriers to access are an essential part of health service responsiveness. Whilst there may be inevitable trade-offs between equality, scarce resources, and efficiency (Nattrass 2004) the fundamental aspect of rights-based equity in health lies in minimizing the presence of *avoidable* health inequalities and barriers to access. Rather than an equal allocation of resources equity implies the allocation of *fair* shares in resources (McCoy 2003). With suggested amendments based on a deeper awareness of context, the right to health framework set out earlier would appear critical to a fairer process.

Decision-making and equity considerations appear to cut across what to do about barriers to access. As suggested earlier, the difficulty in balancing competing principles governing eligibility for ARVs, according to Daniels, adds urgency to the requirement of a "fair process" to air them through public debate and information. Daniels mentions five key principles, of which, one, *stakeholder participation*, is particularly relevant. Daniels' view of participation is that it is aimed at building consensus on rationale to "seek mutually justifiable terms of cooperation"(Daniels 2004:17). This is one interpretation of the role of participation. More generally, the role envisaged for people living with AIDS and community organization participation in HIV/AIDS related policies and programs is considerable. In terms of "3 by 5" itself, specific interpretations, however, tend to fluctuate across related policy documents. In the "3 by 5" document, great scope is suggested for people living with AIDS and community involvement in advocacy, planning, and delivery. There is an implicit understanding that involvement by the community and people living with AIDS will produce more successful responses to HIV/AIDS (WHO 2004a:5). While so central to the "3 by 5" strategy, here, as elsewhere, community involvement can quickly be regarded in much more functional terms, such as providing inputs into program design and management, care, and encouraging adherence (International HIV/AIDS Alliance 2002). In some projects, as well as potentially acting as a buffer to the "development of local patronage or even corrupt practices," McCoy says, "community structures have also been established to ratify and legitimize decisions about patient selection" (McCoy (2003:33). All of this is undoubtedly vital to the success of "3 by 5." Participation is an important principle in rights-based approaches. But it should be promoted whilst also posing more critical questions about what effects participation actually has, including its flaws. I found in some of my previous work during fieldwork in Zambia, when the issue of community participation in selection committees was put to respondents, interestingly, all unanimously rejected it. They did so because they saw it as inherently flawed. It risked recreating prejudiced judgment and exclusion of undesirable patients.

The following chapters seek to give this broader level, deeper context to better understand many of the issues raised surrounding contested meanings of rights, access, criteria, and fair process and accountability. The chapters do this by relating the issues to the experiences of people living with AIDS themselves and key informants. These experiences are inserted into a larger cultural, political, and institutional setting to produce a more comprehensive understanding of "real time" access in Hammanskraal-Temba.

CHAPTER 3

An "Unnatural Place"

Temba/Hammanskraal

> . . . for some strange reason, I always felt that God and the weather [referring to a huge flood in the 1970s in the area] have a tendency to desert a starving and hopeless people right in the middle of their man-made sorrows and political rape.
>
> —Bongani Madondo, a writer from the Temba/Hammanskraal area.[1]

Like many other areas in post-apartheid South Africa, Temba/Hammanskraal (a collective name for, as we shall see, an extensive and diverse geographic area) has been characterized and burdened by its highly complex political, socioeconomic, and cultural geography. Because so much of the transformation post-1994 is directed toward untangling the intricate spatial webs of apartheid era provincial, Bantustan and municipal boundaries, detailing some of this background is important. It will help us to understand how the "man made sorrows and political rape" continue to affect contemporary aspects of service delivery and political dynamics.

Spatial demarcations under apartheid were in particular directed at political and racial ends. The 1959 Bantu Self-Government Act laid the framework for the Bantustans. These were artificially created "states" based upon territorial division, the revival of chieftaincy, and their continuing export of labor to service "white" South Africans. Bantustan political institutions and leadership were created and reinvented as "traditional" mechanisms of Bantu society. This policy was also increasingly linked to efforts to reverse the economic stagnation and collapse of areas, which, following colonialism and the underdevelopment of black farming had functioned as labor reserves. Increasingly, the Bantustans were recast by apartheid South Africa as a "Third World" and "development" problem, particularly to legitimize separating them spatially from "white" areas (Jones 1999). By the late 1960s and early 1970s, the maintenance of white supremacy became linked to developing these peripheral regions as viable entities through a program of modernization. This policy involved massive social engineering and revoking South African citizenship with the forced relocation of millions to the Bantustan margins of "white" South Africa. Temba would be geographically placed in Bophuthatswana, one of four Bantustans, which, with the compliance of their local black leaders, gained "independence" from the apartheid regime in the late 1970s and early 1980s. These states were the Transkei, Venda, Bophuthatswana, and Ciskei Bantustans (henceforth, "TVBC" states). Another six were given self-governing status.

In recent years, the portrayal of supposedly homogenized social relations in the Bantustans has been replaced with a focus upon their local variation. And the image of internal developments in the Bantustans as always subordinate to apartheid and successive apartheid governments in Pretoria is somewhat reappraised. A more dynamic approach had been necessary in order to explore and understand the rapid pace of change within the Bantustan territories (Southall, Segar, and Donaldson 1992). Despite the extreme neocolonial dependency upon the South African state, such a view often ignores the agency of the different political, cultural actors and forces, economic classes, and pseudo state structures given space over many years within the Bantustans. Not least, for over twenty years, residents, in places like Temba, experienced a period of illegitimate, authoritarian institutional and ethnonationalist control during the era of quasi-independent Bophuthatswana. This has left a significant "footprint," as suggested, upon the microgeography of Temba and the institutional structures under its jurisdiction.

The variations within Bantustan social formations led to a politics of state disjuncture between different factions. The fragmentation has been attributed to the differences between the bureaucratic and civil fractions of the petite bourgeoisie in particular. Popular resistance, especially in the 1980s, and the failure of state-led ethnic nationalism to mobilize at the local level were also critical to the collapse of these entities.[2] An important dimension added to these debates has been the character of Bantustan leaders themselves and their discourses of ethnicity and nationalism. Lucas Mangope vigorously imprinted Tswana nationalism upon Bophuthatswana. He also handpicked and micromanaged administrators in the Bophuthatswana state, mainly in order to limit political dissent against his regime. Such was the level of Mangope's intervention that he even personally appointed the management at Jubilee hospital. One local resident who lived in Temba throughout this era described Mangope as a "master of every trade," implying he had a very energetic and versatile role in exercising and maintaining his own political power.[3] As profound an impact as limited resources and poor service delivery were for the area, an additional feature was that inhabitants were denied any form of popularly chosen local governance.

The legacy of Bophuthatswana was therefore vested in the organizational culture of places like Jubilee itself. The chapter explores the interface between the quality of local democracy and delivery of services.

The "nation-building" exercise was therefore bound up with asserting—somewhat ambiguously—both Tswana identity (to be different) and the urgency of escape from the abnormality of being "undeveloped" (in order to become the same), while seeking to maintain political control. The official "spin" of apartheid-era planning described Temba as one of only a few "planned" black towns. The location would be integrally bound to the development of an industrial growth point at Babelegi. These factors would indeed be important determinants of the shape and development of Temba. But much less emphasis in apartheid discourse was given, of course, to Temba's *raison d'etre*—as a repository for all dispossessions, displacements, and evictions from surrounding rural and urban areas deemed "white." Already in the 1940s, according to van Huyssteen, 250 houses were planned, and many of the inhabitants were evicted from either rural or urban areas. These formal houses became the historical core of Temba Township. Martha Ntobeng's[4] family was one of the first in Temba location. Her parents had been subsistence farmers in Limpopo, growing mealies. Encountering immense difficulties to survive, the family migrated to Temba because they thought there would be better chances of employment near Pretoria. Ntobeng's father worked on the railway at Hammanskraal station. Born in 1950, in Temba location, Ntobeng recalls the three-roomed rented house of her parents being one of no more than forty properties. As she grew up, she remembers that a mixture of languages was spoken by her neighbors: Sotho, Sepedi, Zulu, and Tsonga in particular. And contrary to the Tswana nationalist tendencies of the Bantustan regime, this ethnic mix would remain a defiant characteristic feature of Temba. The official languages used at her school were Sotho, English, and Afrikaans.

Rapid change came to the area, not least in the number of houses, which grew quickly to over 3,000 by the end of the 1970s, 90 percent of which was built by the South African Development Trust. The Bophuthatswana era also saw the construction of many four-roomed houses and some electrification of formal areas. Babelegi would also provide employment for residents. However, Ntobeng, like many others, recalls the drudgery for those who worked in "white" Pretoria. The first train left Hammanskraal at 3:00 a.m., with a second at 4:00 a.m. Trains left so early because the journey to Pretoria, although only approximately sixty kilometres away, took more than two and a half hours. During the Bophuthatswana era, bus services would alleviate this hardship to some extent. So, whilst some of these developments in the Bophuthatswana era were welcomed by residents, the underlying spatial, racial, and economic logic of apartheid was never far away: "Mangope tried to make us happy but we were not happy . . . My first job was in a tannery in Babelegi. The work was fine but the problem was the money. We were paid only R6.50 a week. And the law was too tough. They [Bophuthatswana] forced us to do things that we did not want."[5] Places like Temba were overburdened with a growing population incommensurate to its meagre resources.

Another important strand in the area's complex tapestry was a history of disputed land claims. Whereas the land had been predominantly under the control of the Amandebele ba Libalo (Kekana) Tribal Authority, it was increasingly appropriated and excised by various governments. Various ventures included a casino project and the industrial estate at Babelegi. Disputed land claims often resulted in incursions by the same governments into tribal affairs and sowed seeds of dysfunctional governance between the two well into the more recent post-apartheid era.

In the 1980s, the level of political unrest and opposition to apartheid and Bantustan leaders increased. By the early 1990s, with apartheid increasingly unraveling, both economically and politically, Lucas Mangope shifted his political strategy from the construction of Bophuthatswana ethno-"nation"-building characteristic of his rule toward the development of a regionalist coalition of conservative interests. With a finalized constitutional arrangement about to be settled to deliver a unitary South African state, the regime appeared obstinate in the face of transformation. Finally, in 1993, the intransigence in refusing to accept reincorporation into a post-apartheid state saw the regime dramatically swept from power in a popular uprising. Bophuthatswana administrative regions were absorbed primarily into the new North West province. In 1994, the ANC gained overwhelming support in the North West province, winning over 80 percent of the vote in the provincial elections, which Mangope's Bophuthatswana Christian Democratic Party did not contest (Jones 1999). Following the 1999 general elections, which they did contest, Mangope's party, renamed the United Christian Democratic Party, became the largest opposition party in the North West province (but with under 9 percent of the vote). Mangope's political survival probably reflects little more than some limited residual support from former disaffected civil servants, former allies, some traditional leaders, and members of the older generation. Above all, the generous nature of South Africa's proportional representation system for small opposition parties allows three UCDP members to sit as members of Parliament. But the legacy also illustrates a broader set of less formal political issues reflecting the continuing role of interests and identities developed in the Bophuthatswana era. These continue to shape the process of democratic consolidation after 1994. Reincorporated into a unitary state and the transfer and disposal of Bophuthatswana's assets and institutions has been at the center of the complex renegotiations of relations between South Africa's provinces and the central government. More generally, "the inheritance of the homeland lingers like the proverbial albatross, about the new [North West] government" (Seiler 1999). The ANC has been committed to dismantling "islands of apartheid" in the administrative and para-statal structures of the former TVBC states. But this runs up against conservative regional interests, old and new networks of patronage, as well as an ambivalent ANC commitment to the decentralization of power and participatory forms of governance. Developmental efforts post-1994 have therefore sought to unravel these artificial boundaries. Created as expressions of ethnic and racial separation, the aim has been to move from apartheid era boundaries instead to more socially, administratively, and economically logical entities. The logic of the latter, however, would be postponed in the immediate post-apartheid demarcation process. Temba, as noted, had previously been in Bophuthatswana, along with other neighboring areas such as Mabopane, Winterveld, and Ga-Rankuwa. And so-called white Hammanskraal, particularly the "Village Dorpie," where expatriate managers of companies at Babelegi lived, had been adjacent but within then apartheid "white" South Africa. But the demarcation process intended to fix this spatial disharmony actually brought to the surface fissures in the local landscape.

First, lobbying by Tswana nationalists during the demarcation process for the post-apartheid provincial boundaries led to political pressure to keep together as many former Bophuthatswana regions as possible. They wanted to do so by placing them within the newly created North West province, rather than transferring them to Gauteng, as had been originally proposed (Jones 1999).[6] It is, however, important to note that Temba-Hammanskraal residents had shown considerable opposition to the Bophuthatswana regime over the years. The ethnic diversity of the area was a particular provocation to the Tswana nationalists of the Bantustan regime who virulently persecuted the non-Tswana population. This split between the North West and Gauteng would be a particular characteristic of the area (see "The problem of Boundaries").

Second, the residents association of Hammanskraal did not want Mandela Village, a squatter settlement, to be incorporated with it into Gauteng for fear of the financial burden. The local tribal authority also wanted the settlement (now actually largely formalized) in the North West province because it still claimed the territory as its own in spite of the occupation.

The investigating commission determining demarcation of Temba initially appeared to lean toward its inclusion in Gauteng because it was functionally linked to the Pretoria City region. However, they appeared to backtrack, possibly due to broader real politick considerations linked to the multiparty negotiations determining South Africa's post-apartheid settlement. Politicians and planners appeared to force the process. It was declared that these areas be placed under the administration of the North West province, whose capital was the former stronghold of Bophuthatswana, Mafikeng. According to van Huyssteen, this decision was taken "regardless of the pleas by communities and disputes within the demarcation board" (van Huyssteen 2000:10) Temba would therefore lie within the North West's Moretele district, Hammanskraal in Gauteng. The consequences of demarcation have been many and profound, not only for AIDS service but all service delivery.

Realigning Post-apartheid Geography: Pretoria's Peri-urban Fringe

> Hammanskraal is far from important things you understand.
>
> —resident

This demarcation process reflected the creation of provincial boundaries. In 2000, another level, however, involved the demarcation of municipalities. This resulted in a decision to amalgamate many places in former Bophuthatswana areas within the newly formed City of Tshwane (Pretoria) Metropolitan Council, whilst still under provincial jurisdiction of the North West province. This therefore resulted in what are termed "cross-border" municipalities. In effect forming a northern and western peri-urban fringe to Pretoria, the official motivation for the amalgamation was to meet the developmental needs of these disadvantaged areas by including them within the tax base and local economy of a well-serviced conurbation.[7] Undoubtedly, these were important efforts to create geographies of inclusion rather than exclusion. That said, however, a history of complicated boundary configurations, commensurate mixed community affiliations, and socioeconomic deprivation and lack of inclusive local governance inevitably continue to have a profound imprint upon these areas' ability to meet needs.

To that end, the 2000 demarcation process in particular led to the creation of South Africa's first ever-inclusive "wall to wall" municipalities. These gained increasing legitimacy with the 2000 local government elections. Each municipality is now divided into wards with elected ward councilors, ward committees selected from the community, and proportionately allocated council seats.

Collectively, this peri-urban fringe—all those areas mentioned, plus Soshanguve—is now termed "Zone A" in the City of Tshwane and constitutes a quarter of the city region's total population. The differences in development between Zone A and the rest of Pretoria is stark, however. Of "Zone A," more than 74 percent has access to only pit latrines and just 24 percent has access to refuse services of local authority once a week. Furthermore, more than 15 percent rely on access to water supply that is more than 200 meters from the household.[8] Within Temba and Hammanskraal, more specifically, the challenges are no less immense.

Temba/Hammanskraal is a term for what is an extensive geographic area that is often taken by locals and others to mean also several surrounding villages and settlements. For purposes of this book, the geographic, statistical, and political definition of Temba/Hammanskraal will be based primarily upon those wards that form the historical "core" of the area *and*, in addition, the catchment area for Jubilee. The hospital itself is in Ward 74, near Temba location. Definition is therefore based upon Wards 73, 74, 75—the core—as well as wards farther away—8, 76, and some of ward 14 (the eastern part, around Stinkwater) of the City of Tshwane. An additional consideration is that, according to the ARV clinic at Jubilee, many patients come from the Moretele Municipality in the North West province. For example, Mathibistad, a large rural settlement in Moretele, over 20 kilometers away (plus other surrounding areas within the North West province), is considered to constitute the bulk of Jubilee's ARV patients. If we take all these wards (except 14, as much of this would also include population figures for Soshanguve, serviced by another hospital) the total population is approximately 150,000. In addition, 180,000 people live in adjacent Moretele Municipal Authority. On this basis, a review of the 2001 census data for those Tshwane municipality wards comprising Temba/Hammanskraal shows the following key characteristics.

As suggested, the area is extremely ethnically diverse. Although the Setswana-speaking population is the biggest single ethnic group across all wards (except Ward 8), they comprise more than 50 percent of inhabitants in only one ward (Ward 75), and are closely followed numerically by large Sepedi and also Tsonga populations (the latter is largest group in Ward 8), respectively. There are also small, yet significant, Ndebele-, and to a lesser extent, Sotho- and Zulu-speaking communities. Moretele Local Authority, as a whole, is predominantly Tswana-speaking (47 percent) but also has a large Tsonga and Sepedi community. In all wards, the number of "traditional" marriages is almost as high as those classified as "civil," particularly in Ward 8 (44 percent traditional marriages), to a low of 33 percent traditional marriages in Ward 75 (and with a similar "low" for Moretele). These figures therefore reveal that there are cultural practices here that tend to be associated more with rural South Africa. It also has profound developmental challenges.

Development Challenges

The majority of inhabitants in this area were poorly serviced under apartheid, and since 1994, informal settlements have grown considerably. The following developmental challenges are apparent.

Water

The percentage of residents with access to their "own piped water" is between a low of 0.4 percent (Ward 8, which has the largest dependence upon bore-hole water supply) and mainly between 7 to 13 percent for all other wards. The majority, between 36 and 51 percent, across all wards, depend upon the Regional Scheme for water. Between 12 to 32 percent (Ward 74 being lowest, and 73, highest) have water piped in the "yard."

Electricity

Approximately 50 percent of households use electricity for lighting (rising to over 84 percent in Ward 8, and 97 percent in Ward 73), and for cooking, this is less, at around 50 percent, with the lowest being Ward 8 at 30 percent.

Refuse and Sanitation

In terms of refuse service: collection once a week ranges from a low of 30 percent (Ward 8, and 73) to a high of 70 percent (Ward 75), with Ward 74 in between at approximately 50 percent. In terms of access to toilet facilities, the overwhelming majority relies on a pit latrine (89 percent and 92 percent, Wards 8 and 76, respectively), with the notable exception of Ward 75 and 74, where 66 percent and 50 percent, respectively, have their own flush toilets.

Economic Indicators

Economically, all wards (including 76) are characterized by a very high number of those either designated unemployed or not officially active economically. On average this category is approximately 66 percent of residents. The highest number is 72 percent in Ward 8, and the lowest, 59 percent in Ward 75. In terms of earnings, the biggest single group of earners monthly ranges from being most earning under R1600 (Wards 74,73) to R800 (Ward 8). Those classified as earning no income at all: 74 percent (Ward 8) to a low of 21 percent (Ward 73), with Wards 74 and 75 at 25 and 67 percent, respectively.

The area is therefore, in general, "peri-urban" in terms of access to services. But across wards there is unevenness in services, particularly in earning levels. The level deteriorates as one moves further from the township "core" of Temba/Hammanskraal (again, Wards 73, 74, and 75). Wards 8 and 76 appear particularly disadvantaged, reflecting a more rural character. Generally, there appears to be a reasonable degree of access to electricity for lighting but very poor access to water (even in the "core"), and heavy dependence upon pit latrines (with exceptions, as noted, of Ward 74 and 75). In comparison, the Moretele local authority appears to be even more poorly serviced and has a higher percentage of residents (75 percent) classified as not earning; of those who do, the biggest single group earns under R800.

The area's socioeconomic needs are therefore considerable. There is a local needs register called a "Needs register of the previous 5-year cycle" based according to each ward which sheds light on these challenges. This "needs register" was compiled by local government for all of "Zone A," an area including Hammanskraal/Temba and defined by the City of Tshwane Metropolitan Municipality.[9] This reveals, amongst other things, common problems identified, such as illegal dumping and littering. The needs register also indicates the challenges of developing and electrifying the informal settlements in this area. It is of particular interest for the next chapter to note the concerns raised about the local district hospital, Jubilee. The latter is regarded as overstretched because it is also the only hospital serving neighboring Moretele. The need for "cleaning up of Jubilee hospital" was stressed as particularly important (Ward 75). The poor physical condition of Jubilee, including residences for the nursing staff, featured throughout the research period. The long grass was said to conceal snakes and baboons were not an uncommon site. During a local *Imbizo* (that is, a public consultation meeting between decision makers and residents of an area) over the state of the hospital, one irate resident lambasted the poor conditions at Jubilee, claiming "beds were worn out, toilets are not flushing and cockroaches were all over."[10] One implication of this pressure upon the services provided by Jubilee was the excess demand placed upon the local Temba clinic, described as too overcrowded.

In addition, schools are identified as overcrowded and urgently in need of refurbishment and extensions. Facilities are generally needed, including multipurpose centers and high mast lighting (common demands in other wards as well). Crime is also mentioned as a serious issue (Ward 74), so much so that it was causing clinics to shut down at night due to lack of crime prevention measures. Similar issues are identified in terms of demands for general infrastructure improvement, and facilities, and specifically, the need to upgrade pit latrines to water-borne sewerage systems as well as water and electricity supply problems (Ward 73). Another common concern raised was the overflow of sewerage due to faulty pumps. The issue of the "formalization" of informal areas was, unsurprisingly, given the socioeconomic needs identified from the census data, particularly an issue in Ward 8. This included the need for two clinics, and additional schools, housing, sanitation, and running water. These challenges for service delivery, if not already severe, were exacerbated by a particular characteristic of the area: its cross border status and the lingering problem of boundary demarcations.

The Problem of Boundaries

"Demarcation is giving us problems: we want what other people are getting, and most want to go to Gauteng" (SANCO activist, Hammanskraal).

There is a major challenge in creating viable and functional borders. Cross-border governance has impacted greatly upon service delivery (see Figures 3.1 and 3.2). These range from the more minor, yet important, issues, such as responsibility for traffic light maintenance outside of Babelegi industrial estate to more serious service delivery issues. For example, cross-boundary status has had profound consequences for education delivery. The plight of two schools is illustrative of these problems. These schools were recently dubbed "schools of shame" by the print media. In both cases, neither Gauteng nor North West province chose to take responsibility for service provisions and disputed their obligations. As a result, both schools were extremely rundown, with some classrooms without roofs, ceilings, and doors, broken windows, and loose electrical cables. Concerning one, Lethamaga Middle S School, although the state minister for education had expressed shock upon visiting the school in 2005,

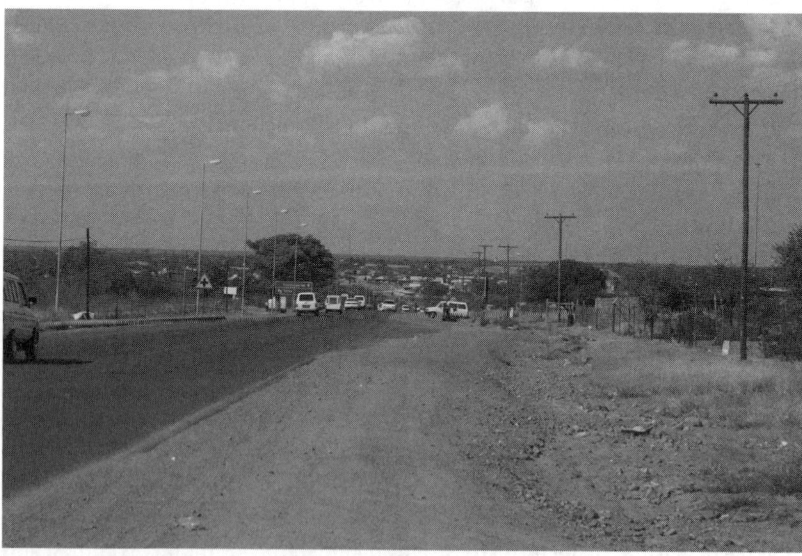

Figure 3.1 Hammanskraal to Soshanguve Road

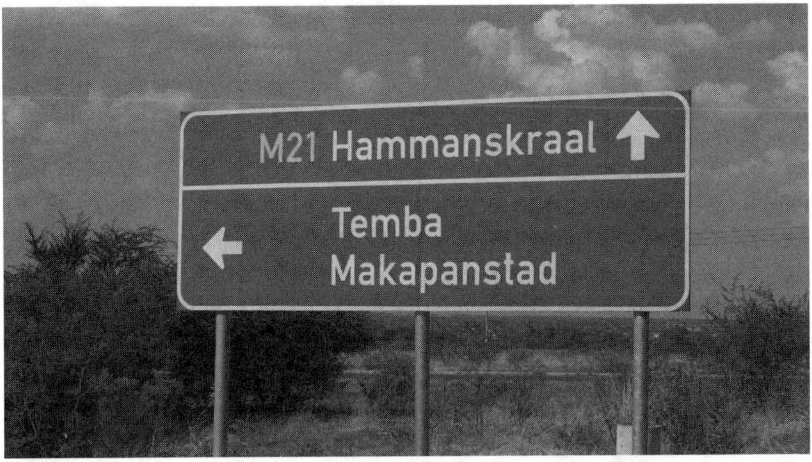

Figure 3.2 Places on the Edge

no improvements had been made even by the start of 2007. It was claimed by the principal that this was because he had been informed that "the North West government was not prepared to spend money on a school that would be [soon] part of Gauteng."[11] The government had decided to finally end cross-border jurisdictions. But in interviews and group discussions, it appears that there has been inadequate preparation for transfer of services to Gauteng. In terms of the hospital, local COSATU representatives claimed that some payments accruing to staff had been withheld due to the impending transfer to Gauteng.[12] Management was identified as responsible for delaying payments, with little preparation for transfer and a lack of transparency, tending to fuel interpretations apparently that "everything is corrupt" prior to transfer to Gauteng. In another instance, a home-based care organization based in Marokolong (in Ward 73, between the R101 road and N1 highway) described how they were facing a new era in having to make new contacts with Gauteng social and health services based in Tshwane. They viewed this with great trepidation, having been accustomed to the North West institutional structures. Again, there appeared to be no preparation for transfer. And with critical shortages in home-based care kits, and the need to get more food parcels and school uniforms for distribution to clients, the uncertainty was proving stressful for the leadership (of Perseverance Rural Development Centre).[13]

Other instances of problems related to boundaries involved the impact on crime prevention efforts. For example, a study in 2003 found that cross-border service delivery concerning crime prevention was hampered. Performance of functions was difficult, for example, because there was poor coordination between the South Africa Police Service and the metropolitan police. In addition, collecting and processing crime statistics by different provinces and competing provincial priorities and legislation were compounding issues. Even the availability of a (toll-free) number to report crime was an issue because while it was available in Pretoria, it was not in Temba.[14] In some instances, cross-border problems reinforced inequality in, or perceptions of, unequal access to services. On a fundamental level, residents and service providers were sometimes unable to agree where borders—and hence responsibilities—ended or began. The impact upon health services has been similarly serious. Provincial allocation of resources depends upon calculations of the number of residents of a province utilizing those services, whilst users from other provinces would warrant charging that province (Palmary and Ngubeni 2000).[15] And there is increasing anecdotal evidence to suggest that since the transfer of Jubilee to Gauteng, some patients living in North West Province have been refused treatment at the hospital.

In 2005, the confused spatial imprint upon health service delivery appeared to reach its zenith of madness with the delay in rollout of ARV drugs at Jubilee in the North West province. Journalist Henk Rossouw in particular captures the effect of geography and why it is especially seared upon this location:

> In the Winter of 2005, the hospital [Jubilee] had access to drugs but, without government accreditation, had n't managed to give them out yet. For over a year treatment had been available in certain hospitals in Gauteng . . . whose boundary enclosed the capital city of Pretoria. He [the doctor in question] had already pleaded with hospitals in Gauteng to allow patients to cross the boundary and get treatment in the city but they had refused; they had their own queue and his patients lived outside of their jurisdiction. The district hospital is in the North West province and falls short of being part of Gauteng by a millimetre, the width of a fence. On provincial maps, the boundary is literally the hospital's southern fence. Most mornings, on his way to the clinic, Robinson [the pseudonym given to the doctor] drove across the boundary line between living and dying (Rossouw 2006).

The quotation above powerfully captures the stark nature of the twin challenges confronting Hammanskraal/Temba, namely, service delivery and, with the area's cross-border status, the associated burden of geography. These vivid constraints serve to highlight how issues surrounding availability of drugs, and their cost and supply, should be placed within a broader context that constitutes *access*. There are several additional important political features that interface with access to ARV services and, indeed, the more general issue of service delivery.

Locating Accountability

Limited residual support for the UCDP (previously named, as mentioned, the Bophuthatswana Christian Democratic Party) has been eclipsed by widespread popular support for the ruling ANC party in the area. That support for the ANC, based on the 2006 local election results,[16] ranges from a high of 93 percent (Ward 8), followed by 91 percent (Ward 73), 89 percent (Ward 76), 80 percent (Ward 75), to a "low" of 78 percent (Ward 74). The only apparent significant challenge from other political parties is around 6 percent from the UCDP and the Democratic Alliance in Ward 75. The highest ward vote for a "runner-up" is in fact from independent candidates—at 9 percent in Ward 4—whose showing was bigger than any of the official opposition parties across *all* wards. Moretele also has an overwhelming ANC majority, with 87 percent voting for party in the 2006 local elections.

There are at least three powerful dynamics structuring, and also structured by, local politics relations. One dynamic concerns that of independent candidates standing in local elections, linked to specific issues and ideologies that often cause a split within local ANC structures. But more often than not, in areas like Temba, the emergence of independents appears correlated with the politics of patronage. That is, these independents generally tend to be on the "losing side" of patronage, namely, they are sidelined from the governing structures and hence stand independently. As a local SANCO leader expressed it, these independents "are not in the family any more," that is, the ruling ANC.[17] Reasons given for their exclusion from ruling networks include their apparent criticism of existing patronage, and perhaps a desire to expose corrupt practices, or, it may be because they perceive themselves not to be benefiting from the spoils. For each, the outcome is similar—they are no longer privy to the award of council and other government tenders, known as "CC" or "Close Cooperation" agreements. These CCs are particularly significant because they are material resources, like contracts for building houses. A spur to leaving the ANC was suggested in that these tenders are awarded "because I know you," in other words, you are a party loyalist or a family member or, perhaps, both. But to what extent is local government itself known to the average resident outside of these networks?

A second dynamic therefore concerns the generally poor relations between municipalities, councilors, and residents. In 2004, research from the Tswelopele project revealed that most members of the local social clubs interviewed regarded the local government and ward councilors as being of little consequence, or, having little impact on the lives of the community. There were often complaints that the councilors only appeared during elections, and soon after disappeared, failing to deliver on promises made. Consistent themes in responses were the identification of problems associated with roads, housing, water, and other basic services. Residents suggested that councilors were too preoccupied with nurturing their own patronage-based support. Local government councilors also identified the issue of slow development as a major concern but cited as causes the presence of traditional leaders, the fact that the area was relatively new and that huge backlogs existed. Councilors said that they had a good relationship with the cross-border municipality, and that there was sharing on certain projects. However, there was no budget sharing to reflect this. And the poor image of councilors is exacerbated in recent years as many choose to live in former 'white' areas rather than locally.

A third characteristic is that given the distance between local government and residents, particular importance should appear to be attached to encouraging more participatory governance and decision-making. However, it became apparent that supposedly consultative meetings, more often than not, are usually predetermined, with issues and participants preselected rather than genuinely participatory. Participation, more generally, tends to favor more organized and better-resourced groups (Friedman 2006). Throughout South Africa, there is emerging evidence that the majority of the structures created to embolden local democracy—ward committees—are failing to live up to expectations. In one example, the aims stated as to enhance participation in municipality "Integrated Development Plans" and to discuss and prioritize local community needs and municipal development appears contrary to the reality. In South Africa's biggest city, the strategic agenda and indicative budget allocations were in fact agreed five months *before* consultation with citizens. Not only does this reflect how participation is often predetermined rather than genuine, but additionally that the draft IDP was not even shared with ward committees appears to confirm their peripheral role in local policy making and participation.[18]

Some local residents in Temba went further in this criticism, suggesting that the ward committees themselves have become nothing other than vehicles of patronage and enrichment. Although representation appeared at face value to draw upon the strengths of different sectors, one respondent observed how the motivation to join the committee (by being selected by the ward councilor) was "to get bread"; that is, for personal financial gain. This was apparent in positioning for tenders for contracts unrelated to the representative's sectoral specialism and in establishing organizations to get tenders rather than involving already existing organizations with expertise. One of the other flaws was the apparent lack of reporting back to the community. The existing chair of the ward committee's position was allegedly related more to his ANC activism rather than qualifications. This seems to be illustrative of a lack of transparency in recruitment. The phrase "redeployment" captures the award of positions due to party loyalty rather than merit or skills. This, together with favorable access to tenders for infrastructural development, produces, as suggested in Chapter 1, also nationally, an overlapping Gordian knot of economic and political interests. The tendency not to advertise local employment opportunities in local council and even to give preference to family members[19] is also related to lack of transparency. It was claimed that it is also commonplace not to advertise tenders. Often, councilors have already chosen recipients before they consult—and even if they do actually consult—the community. The uneven standards of service and accountability in this area are illustrated in the following contrasting examples.

A group discussion held with people living with AIDS and home-based carers in Stinkwater revealed that one of the biggest issues for those receiving ARV treatment in areas like this is the sheer distance involved in accessing it at Jubilee (see Chapter 7).[20] It was attended by half a dozen female people living with AIDS, and up to four carers from a community care organization. When asked what would make access and adherence easier, it is unsurprising that the people living with AIDS made requests for a mobile clinic. They turned to the home-based carers present at the meeting in an appeal for support in this endeavor. Almost as quickly in response, however, one of the male carers at the back of the small room responded tersely that "there is a ward committee and councilor and protocol which alone dictates bringing services here." Observing the exchange in the wind-swept RDP house where the meeting took place seemed indicative of a set of distances circumscribing access to ARVs. It certainly captured the distance between these people living with AIDS and their professed carers, a perception reinforced by their respective body language and physical separation at the meeting. But it also revealed their distance from formal political processes in the local area. And, in so far as these very same processes—or "protocols"—serve to channel issues, they act as a form of political control by the patronage machine sidelining citizens.

In contrast, for another resident, her experience of dealing with local councilors is very different.[21] For her, the issue of municipal-led cleaning policy was cited as a particular problem because neighbors apparently dump refuse on whatever open land is available. But in terms of getting some accountability in rectifying this, in contrast to the people-living-with-AIDS group, this resident is able to directly phone her local councilor, Mr. Mahlangu. When he is not available, the resident is able leave phone messages on voice mail, to which she says Mahlangu responds. On one occasion, she recalled how the councilor personally came to her home and showed her the account books, which indicated that while some people were paying dues (rates levies), many more did not. This meant that only a certain amount of money was available for cleaning and that the budget had to be stretched over a wide area. Whereas the majority of residents spoke in common about disappointing feedback from local politicians, this resident regarded the response as exhibiting good governance.[22] Why should there be two such different standards for accountability? Why should the resident in question, who is a middle-aged, white female and by no means partisan to liberation politics, be able to command such a response when so many others claim their communities never see councilors? Could one explanation be that because they are practically neighbors in the upper income housing section of Hammanskraal (the "Village Dorpie") that the defining feature for accountability in this case is class based? The councilor in question himself has his own private house there, as well as two guesthouses for paying guests. This probably enables a greater chance of face-to-face contact than would otherwise be facilitated by a patronage network. But it does represent a conundrum that challenges one-dimensional explanations of political development in South Africa: whilst service delivery is de-democratizing for the majority in this area, paradoxically, it appears democratizing for others. To what extent can rights seek to fill this apparent gap in accountability?

Local Perceptions of Rights

The understanding and use of human rights in this local community reflects an acute disjuncture between "global" (and "national" rights) talk and local meanings of rights. In Hammanskraal and Temba, it was clear from both earlier and more recent research that the human rights approach to HIV/AIDS had not been effective at community level. All those ideals espoused in international and national guidelines and policies, and the rights contained in the (national) Bill of Rights and other protective legislation had simply not permeated down to community level. When asked about the Constitution and the Bill of Rights, the majority of people interviewed were able only to recognize them but not give any details on what was in them. Questions on the Bill of Rights were met with silence or vague answers about rights, not what those rights entailed in a practical sense. At that stage, there had been little in terms of dissemination of the content at community level. This impacted on people's ability to claim their rights—if a person did not know what they were, they would not be in a position to recognize human rights violations and claim enforcement of rights. There were also discrepancies between knowing about rights and then actually being able to exercise them. But over and above issues to do with information and lack of organizations working on rights, there are fundamentally divergent conceptions and "world views" of rights, as follows. A local traditional leader, Chief Nawa, of *Lebotlaone* (a group of villages of approximately 20,000 people), when asked about the Bill of Rights identified it as eroding the traditional way of life and breakdown of values in the villages. Consider the following exchange:

Interviewer: Okay. What about the Bill of Rights? The Human Rights?
Nawa: Wow.
Interviewer: Have you seen that?
Nawa: (*Laughs*). Jessus. Hey!
Interviewer: Is it good or is it bad?
Nawa: Well, it's bad.
Interviewer: Is it?
Nawa: Yes.
Interviewer: Why?
Nawa: It's bad because it gives the women more power than the men. And eh, the man is the head of the house. But now they are equal. Even if your wife says, "I don't want to cook," you don't want to cook.
Interviewer: Yes.
Nawa: If you try to maybe go to the police they come and arrest you. You see, there's no chance [of maintaining male advantages].
Interviewer: Okay. So you think it's disrupting the . . .
Nawa: . . . the villages.
Interviewer: Okay. Are you finding situations where wives and husbands are having problems because women are saying, "no I'm not doing this and that?"
Nawa: Maybe sometimes . . . a man comes who says I want to sleep with my wife but they don't want to. They say wait for me 'til 3, 2 months.[23]

Here, in this exchange, a traditional leader captures some of the sentiments more generally held by men who fear challenges to masculinity. Part of this lies, especially in this exchange, in the perception that the rights of women now trump other older, traditional, moral or religious values. These rights are now apparently circumventing established norms of dealing with sexuality, such as, according to interview with Nawa, legitimizing hitting a wife to settle a domestic dispute. Most notably, it is therefore implied that gender equality is damaging gender roles that are based on established sexual norms. Indeed, the post-apartheid liberal democratic norms enshrined in the Constitution confer, following Posel, "a stability and authority attached to these new rights, which (in theory) renders them unassailable" to alternative values (Posel 2005:129). Now when men seek to assert themselves, particularly, as above, sexually, this is interpreted as being challenged by top-down liberal values. The reference to the "police may come" possibly indicates the role of special police units to deal with rape and sexual violence. At the very least, it highlights how the era of rights and responsibilities and government obligations has pried open the domestic sphere of sexuality and sexual relations to make them now public matters. As such, the exchange above reveals some of the anxieties and contested views associated with constitutionally enshrined rights.

In considering the power of the Constitution more generally, in this, the challenge posed by municipal councilors was also considered by the traditional leader as part of the disruption of traditional authority. The chief also identified the Local AIDS Council (LAC) as belonging to the municipal council, and hence, implied that there was a similarly poor relationship with it (see the next chapter for LAC). Local government councilors reciprocated by arguing that the rights in the Constitution accorded to traditional leaders were in fact a problem for development of the area. Other state employees, such as a local district health promotion office, referred to traditional leaders as "unhelpful."

Otherwise, some people living with AIDS alleged that access to information for young people made them more likely to engage in sexual behavior, thus leading to a faster spread of HIV. Furthermore, some nurses in this community alleged that access to child-care grants made young women fall pregnant to gain access to money.

Male social clubs alleged that there was a misuse of the freedom of speech, where children had too many rights compared to their parents, and that was why they were able to engage in sex and their parents were unable to comment on their behavior.

Many people suggested that those core features of a rights-based approach to AIDS—confidentiality and informed consent—were unimportant and that nonconsensual HIV testing should take place. More worrisome was some respondents actually identified the emphasis upon privacy and confidentiality as facilitating the spread of HIV/AIDS in the community.[24] One even advocated forcing people into the local stadium and forcibly testing them in order to know their HIV status.

Some other considerations are the sheer amount of time required in actually invoking rights, even presuming the person in question has the social or political capital to do so. Gertrude, a social worker, for example, suggested that claiming rights in a context of poverty, deprivation, and illness was extremely difficult. She cited the example of people appearing to consent to testing when in fact they were doing so not out of empowerment but because of disempowerment through being sick, ill, and lacking confidence. Even for educated people, she (Gertrude) suggested it would be doubtful for them to claim rights: "Why I'm asking is because even if you are uneducated, myself I'm employed. But at home I am also taking care of so many people. This rights issue is not an issue for me. Or even if it is an issue, I'm not in a position to address it as I should because I have to work . . . I have so many dependents, I have to work. So if I have to prioritize, taking leave to address the rights issue, seriously, I won't be able to do it you see?"[25] Finally, the local police tended to see the Bill of Rights as preventing them from doing their jobs properly, and argued that education provided to the community about the 1994 constitution did not include educating people about the accompanying responsibilities.

All of these reflections appear to be far away from global level policy definitions and "gold standard" rights-based standards. Rights, furthermore, also need to negotiate political culture.

The ANC had delivered a constitution and political settlement strongly rooted in human rights, social justice, and equality. However, because there is no viable alternative to the ANC's agenda of transformation, people expressed fear that if they do not vote ANC they will lose out, for example, in terms of grants for children or pensions for old people. The political culture reflects a fundamental misunderstanding that a debt is unconditionally paid to the ANC because of the liberation struggle, rather than focusing on citizenship, institutions, and democratic practice associated with being rights-holders. While the voting pattern undoubtedly and overwhelmingly reflects the position that local people firmly believe the ANC should be ruling, it became apparent that many locals also want to be able to determine who their own leaders are and have a desire to influence and have accountability over them. This tendency toward de-democratization is also related to how little political party competition exists, as mentioned, in the area.

In terms of formal politics, there is slightly higher opposition in certain polling areas, mainly from independent candidates. It is very difficult to correlate voting patterns with level of services in each ward mainly because the socioeconomic data is from 2001 and will not reflect possible changes between then and the local elections in 2006. If voting results are disaggregated around specific polling stations, some show a slightly higher percentage of opposition votes but still only receiving a high of 20 percent at one poll within Ward 74, and 17 percent within one poll in Ward 75. Another trend is the poor level of voter-turnout in the last local election. This ranges from a high of 49 percent in Ward 73, followed by 43 percent in Ward 8, 40 percent Ward 74, to the lowest of 35 percent in Ward 75. So, homogeneous in terms of formal politics and the considerable socioeconomic challenges, the main political dynamics tend to revolve around the inner ANC party and alliance structures, such as SANCO.

One respondent explained why he thought it took so long to get services in his area, Kanana.[26] This, he suggested, was related to a fundamental lack of accountability. For example, the officials would get the budget and then they would allegedly invest it to earn interest rather than using it to deliver services.

Whereas in one area it has taken over a decade for signs of delivery, during ward committee meetings it became apparent that councilors might inform that the work had been contracted but without delivery taking place. Residents are not told why the budget may be "reallocated" for something else. Furthermore, in addition to the lack of scrutiny, the more overt benefits of being in the patronage system—such as the award of tenders mentioned and kickbacks—as well as more general influence over allocation of housing and associated resources, inevitably impacts service delivery. These features appear to be replicated across hundreds of communities throughout South Africa. Information is deliberately withheld by council officials or is not shared with communities. Accordingly, "for a number of communities, they are trying to get the most basic documents, like IDPs, budgets and policy documents."[27] Not getting this and being able to voice concerns adds to local frustrations. So, beyond formal politics, and, indeed, perhaps because of it and its co-opted, constricted, and controlled channels, one of the principal mechanisms for expressing grievances over service delivery has been through protest.

"Chowing Money": Service Delivery Protests in the Area

Chapter 1 mentioned that service delivery protests have been common sites across the country. The North West province has been particularly badly affected. And residents in Hammanskraal and Temba have also consistently expressed frustration with service delivery over the last three years. In terms of one of the dynamics in protests appearing to be the perception of corruption within local authorities (Chapter 1), local residents have made numerous allegations that councilors are corrupt and that they are using resources for their own ends. These practices are described locally as "chowing money." More high-profile cases include the mayor of Moretele municipality, Asnath Molekwa. She apparently used unapproved council funds to pay R400,000 for a car; R150,000 for her inauguration; withheld information from opposition councilors; and was accused of using three bodyguards rather than the one to which she was entitled.[28] Opposition parties claimed that there was a distinct lack of transparency in these dealings. There was also evidence that the budget was overspent without authorization and contracts awarded without being honored. Areas close by to Temba, such as Soshanguve and Winterveld, have boiled over into outright protest. And even closer, in New Eersterus, an informal settlement between Hammanskraal and Soshanguve, 500 residents fought battles with police over poor services.[29] The reason given for the lack of protests in Temba and Hammanskraal was apparently that local mechanisms, no matter how imperfect, did exist to channel frustrations. And, since the 2001 census figures, it is apparent in repeated visits to the area that formalization of services—such

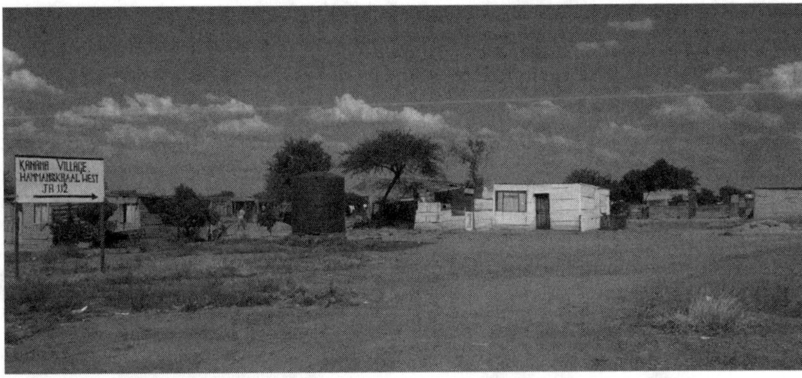

Figure 3.3 Kanana before service delivery

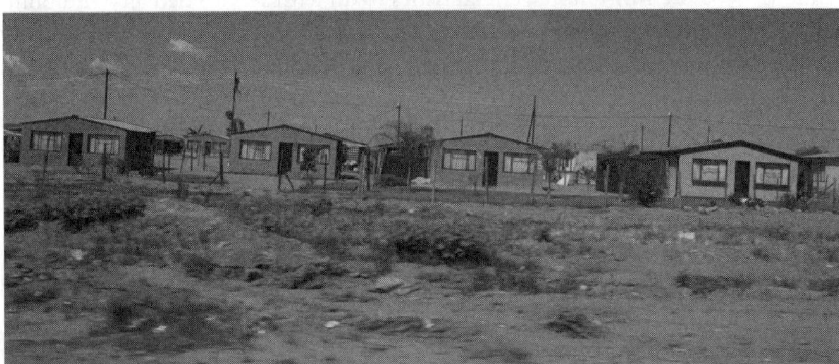

Figure 3.4 Parts of Kanana after RDP house building

as housing, lighting, and water—has slowly taken place over three years, particularly in former squatter areas such as Mandela Village and now Kanana. Slow and strewn with corrupt practices, nonetheless, protest has generally not taken place because delivery is perceived as progressing. But Kanana is still very uneven (see Figures 3.3 and 3.4). But at an *Imbizo* meeting, accusations were directed at local councilors, who, it was claimed, allocated houses to "unlawful beneficiaries."[30]

In April 2007, all these underlying frustrations appeared to finally boil over for some residents. Angry residents in Kanana erupted into fury after being given eviction orders to vacate RDP houses. What ensued, those staples of South African service delivery protests—burning tires, rock throwing, and standoffs with police—adorned the main road from Hammanskraal to Soshanguve opposite Kanana itself. Apparently, many of these residents had paid some local political leaders up to R6000 to occupy these properties, flouting waiting lists and proper procedure for allocation, and hence lacking legality. Such queue-jumping is certainly unfair to those who had been lawfully waiting. Indeed, the housing policy is an area of considerable lack of transparency to do with allocation of houses and also tendering process. Local politicians were even implicated in commandeering cement for their own purposes. Then, in August of the same year, it was the turn of residents in Kanana's shack settlements to vent their own fury due to an eviction order that granted the police permission to forcibly remove residents. This troubled settlement represents something of a microcosm of the nationwide disgruntlement with the path of service delivery and development.[31]

All this is stated because it sketches a background to remind us that it would be naïve to think that institutional structures, like the district hospital, Jubilee, could be separate from more general issues to do with service delivery and political accountability in this community. A variety of difficult challenges confront service delivery. These challenges are next looked at in more detail in relation to the governance of ARV treatment in Hammanskraal/Temba.

CHAPTER 4

"Gambling on Treatment"

Governing ARV Programs

> . . . there are some institutions [like Jubilee] whereby you can't even meet with management, you see. They will say, "no we don't want to meet with you, we are the ones, we are the bosses here, you see." Now, how are you going to deal with issues with such kind of management?
>
> —COSATU, area representative[1]

The broader challenges associated with service delivery in South Africa are often missing in analyses of access to public sector ARV programs. Most commonly, and as important as they inevitably are, access is being gauged according to human resource issues and also individual patient behavior and retention. This chapter therefore locates "access" within the institutional landscape itself to look at how the organizational culture conditions access for people living with AIDS. Not least, this is because ARV clinics have been newly established at a number of district hospitals. These new structures have to interact with broader hospital management and working practices. The bigger administrative picture therefore has a bearing upon how ARV clinics operate. And, on top of this already complex coexistence, is the fact that the ARV issue has been so politicized in South Africa. It is therefore pertinent to ask how such governance issues have shaped the availability and quality of hospital-based care and treatment. Above all, the role of people-living-with-AIDS' own experiences at these institutions, their perceptions of access to AIDS-related services at *Jubilee*, the local hospital, inevitably has a bearing upon how they may seek ARV services. The chapter begins with the story of "T," a person living with AIDS in the area, to illustrate how these issues are integral to unpacking the issue of "access" to ARVs.

"T"'s story

I first met "T" in 2004 at a local support group meeting at a hospice. At that time, "T" had developed full-blown AIDS. I vividly remember his painfully thin frame, his languid movements, and that he was constantly thirsty and swigging water from a plastic container. Strongly opinionated in meetings, his pent-up frustrations appeared to belie some underlying painful experiences. In a focus group, "T" shared some of these experiences. He talked about his late partner's AIDS-related illness. He revealed how the partner's entire family had treated her in a very harsh manner: not caring for her and leaving her alone even when she was terminally ill. He recalled that on one occasion, his partner's grandmother, upon overhearing T's partner talking to someone, shouted out loudly, "why are you talking—I thought you were dead!" This attitude of life having already ended, of stigma and witnessing such exclusion it induces had been particularly painful for "T," as for many others. He also regarded it as a contributory factor in hastening his partner's death. Later, after other encounters, I got to know "T" and spoke with him in more detail.

It soon became apparent that in addition to the loss of his partner, soon after followed the death of their daughter to an AIDS-related condition. And superimposed on the personal experience of loss of loved ones was the added burden of the fear and exclusion generated by family and community members. In 1999, fearing his own deteriorating health was also related to AIDS, "T" tested at clinics and general practitioners several times. Through fear about the implications of discovering his positive status, he had not asked for the results. Finally, upon the insistence of a doctor, "T" attended Jubilee, where his blood was drawn for an HIV test without consent. The harrowing experience—that of someone already vulnerable, fearful, and experiencing loss of loved ones—and hearing negative things about ARVs and being told by a nurse not only that he was positive but that he should "go home and die," inevitably conditioned for "T" what "access" to ARVs meant. When finally made available in the public sector, these painful experiences indelibly shaped access as now something akin to a "gamble": "It was gamble. Actually I put my life at stake. Because I didn't know exactly [whether] the ARVs was gonna help me or is going to make my condition worst. I said it is better I put my life at stake as I have put my life at stake before: because before I realized that I'm HIV positive, then they took my blood [at Jubilee] without my consent. They took blood and then they told me that 'go and die.' You see. So I risk again for going for ARVs."

The experience and perception of "gambling" shapes access to ARVs. First, "T"'s experience of abusive treatment by health care workers and disregard for his status inevitably broke trust and confidence in AIDS-services at the hospital. And the apparent lack of accountability and recourse is germane to service delivery issues more generally. But in addition, compounding this was the deficit of information upon which to inform choices. And that deficit—which the next chapter looks at—is also itself compounded by community-based attitudes to AIDS and ARVs. It is the notion of the insecurities associated with ARVs—or, in "T"'s phrase, "gambling"—which lies at the core of what follows and surely must challenge rational individual models of treatment behavior. "T" did commence ARVs in 2005, but not at Jubilee. In light of the discrimination encountered at the hospital, he preferred to travel much further and at greater cost to a neighboring hospital. Currently, although his health has clearly improved, "T"'s CD4 count still remains stubbornly low. "T"'s last job had been in 1992 as a kitchen fitter for a company at the Babelegi Industrial site. His entire household is now dependent upon "T"'s disability grant. Termination of the grant would clearly have a devastating impact upon both his and the family's efforts to maintain their health. More recently, "T" has been influential in an advocacy group formed in the area (see Conclusion) to contest violations of rights at Jubilee and elsewhere in the community.

Jubilee Hospital and Quality of Care Issues

Jubilee is a district hospital that from 1994 was administered under the North West province, until its transfer to Gauteng in April 2007.

ARV services began at the Wellness clinic, Jubilee, with the initiation of treatment only in September 2005. Since initiation of ARV treatment began,

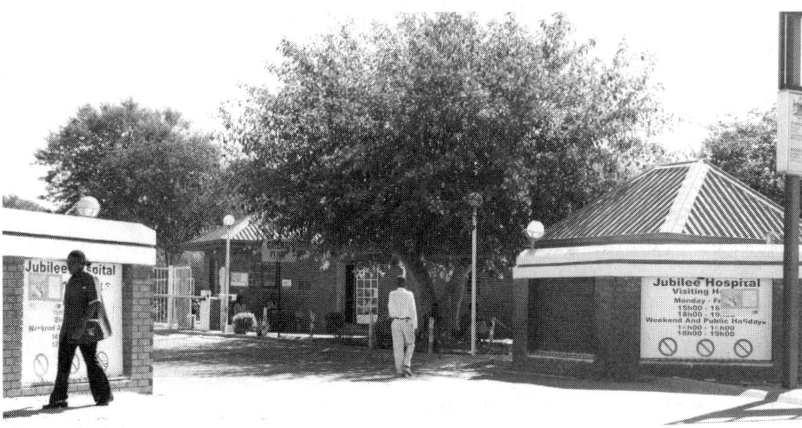

Figure 4.1 Jubilee hospital

Table 4.1 Patient numbers at Wellness clinic, Jubilee hospital

	March 2006	*January 2007*
On Treatment	300	1189
Registered	1000	2500
Waiting	700	1200
Average CD4 count	75	100

the rapid change in patient numbers at the Wellness clinic can be compared over the two time periods during the fieldwork in the "ARV era."

Data is extremely difficult to come by at the clinic level. While I was unable to obtain hard data, in discussions with clinic staff, however, the following breakdown was observed. First, the ratio of female to male patients appears to be approximately 60 percent to 40 percent. Clinic staff identified as particularly problematic the lack of men coming forward for treatment. Second, approximately 10 percent of patients are children. Third, and reflecting socioeconomic context, the majority of patients do not work. They are given nutritional substitutes due to food insecurity. Fourth, despite high numbers of foreigners in the area, they are totally underrepresented at the clinic because they are effectively excluded from access due to nonresidency status. The exclusion was verified by information from the clinic head, who even showed me a directive issued from the North West government to do so for nonresidents. There has therefore been a dramatic increase in ARV patient numbers, almost quadrupling, as well as an almost doubling in size of waiting lists. These rapid changes inevitably produce significant challenges for the clinic and hospital under which it is governed.

Yet, it is with concern, therefore, to note that the first phase of research into stigma and discrimination in the area implicated the hospital consistently and notoriously in the responses of people living with AIDS (Zuberi et al 2004). Indeed, the clear majority of responses across groups of people living with AIDS and also those not living with HIV or AIDS indicated widespread dissatisfaction with health services at Jubilee. Such dissatisfaction can also be located in a broader historical time period. Built in the 1960s, and under management of a Baptist mission, poor services have long been associated with Jubilee and reflect the more general neglect of rural health care in particular. According to one resident, the quality of service did improve during the Bophuthatswana era, with more nurses and shorter waiting times that were also generally on time if you wished to see a doctor. Good care and also medication were apparently "always" available.[2] The quality appears to have declined since 1994.

These resident views are confirmed by studies of the restructuring of national health. Many of these reveal that since 1994, there has been a decline in hospital staff numbers, including, critically, a sharp decline in the number of nurses, and prioritization of strengthening of primary health care (von Holdt and Murphy 2007; Schneider, Barron, and Fonn 2007). In qualitative terms, one of the biggest differences noted, according to locals like long-term resident Martha Ntobeng, is the profound sense of changes in attitudes of nursing staff. Whereas previously, nurses commanded great respect and were well liked, now, apparently "people are only working just to get money," in other words, rather than prioritizing caring. According to Ntobeng, apparently, even when the nurses can see that a person is critical, they will still take their time before attending to the patient. Additionally, medication is also scarcer.

These observations, made by a person born in the area in 1950, also chime with the complaints raised by other people not living with AIDS in focus groups concerning the waiting period, that there were no doctors available and that the drugs were never in the pharmacy. They were generally dissatisfied with the treatment that they received when visiting the hospital. As one female social club member said about being ill and having to go to hospital: "I won't go there, I will stay away."

Many people living with AIDS recounted their own stories, of nurses forcing them to wait to go to the bathroom, being told to "go yourself," gossiping about patients in front of others, passing "funny remarks," and even being refused treatment. Getting the wrong medication and also being placed in specific "HIV" wards were additional issues. But it is the oft-cited tendency to be neglected that is particularly troubling for people living with AIDS: "Sometimes when you are taken to the hospital and they [nursing sisters] can see that you are very ill, they don't attend to you, they just say 'take this person there, there is nothing we can do for him.' They don't want to understand that this person is in pains and needs urgent help, therefore they must give him the special attention; they just become harsh to him. I don't know why they do that. Sometimes they send that sick person back home. So, if a nursing sister tells you to go back home it becomes tough" (unnamed resident).[3]

In many cases, even if very ill, people living with AIDS also said they would prefer to be cared for at home rather than going to Jubilee. One even said they would prefer to die at home than ever go to Jubilee. Although the inadequate care cited appeared generalized also to people not living with AIDS, specific AIDS-related discriminatory practices were common. These included disclosure of status through gossiping or an AIDS-signifying code written on a patient's file. There were therefore violations of privacy and confidentiality and also inadequate information in relation to testing procedures. People living with AIDS also felt aggrieved that there was no mechanism or focal point for seeking redress (see section "Access, Quality, and Care" and Conclusion). They alleged that it was useless to complain since the suggestion boxes that were at the hospital were opened and the suggestions reviewed by the clinics supervisors themselves, who simply removed all complaints. And, according to a former hospital board representative who has since become chair, in his previous capacity, he would compile a report concerning patient complaints. Although this would be discussed, it was, according to him, done so in a very defensive manner, which did not allow for thorough discussion and was therefore ineffective. The last point relates to broader issues in lack of accountability and poor management regarding services that the chapter will return to.

Quality of care issues seem to implicate governance of the hospital more generally. This starts with the most elementary but perhaps one of the most important entry points to the hospital—the role of negotiating hospital clerks: "They [People living with AIDS] are afraid to go back [to the hospital], because then they are having problems as far as the clerks is concerned. When you go to the clinic the clerk is supposed to give you the file. Instead of giving you the file they go through the file, reading what is inside your file. And then after realizing that they are HIV positive, maybe you're staying in the same community, but that very particular clerk gossips about my status" ("T"). The implication was that this behavior impacts upon the people's confidence in whether to go back to Jubilee, with "people . . . afraid to go to the clinic . . . they throw the medication away . . . " Patients at Wellness were acutely aware of the problems in negotiating care and treatment on wards outside the clinic: "The problem is the link between the hospital and the Wellness. There should be correlations you see, between the hospital and the Wellness. That is a problem. We are being send to ward 2 or ward 3 you know we are just an alien" ("Florence"). Accounts of mistreatment by nurses at the hospital were, unfortunately, all too common:

> I went to Jubilee very angry after seeing how they are careless about the patients. They do not even accompany people at hospital but let them go alone. The doctor then said to this one [nurse] (who was making the bed) 'why are you not helping the sick lady?' My heart was so broken. I kneeled down and prayed. This person could not stand up from bed, its difficult for someone to just put her on the chair. When the other one was busy making the beds no one checked the sick one. She even fell down. Jubilee is not a good hospital" (Florence).

Another respondent also said that "Jubilee is not a hospital." She detailed the story of her four-year-old child. After a fall and having internal bleeding and bruising, the mother took the child to Jubilee, where, apparently, the nurses were both judgmental and negligent:

> They [the nurses] shouted at me saying that I do not take care of the child when I asked them for help. The doctor said they are not working but they spend time

> playing cards. I was really crying because of the way they treated my child, only to find that my child has hemophilia. I stayed there for long and they did not help me. They later gave him Panado (paracetomal). Finally, they transferred me to Ga-Rankuwa [another hospital] and when I got there I was asked why I took so long, why was I waiting. I told them. They said that the nurses at Jubilee should have taken my child for blood test and they had not. My child got treated at Ga-Rankuwa. Jubilee, I never want to see it" ("Wandi").

Others recounted their observations of the mistreatment of patients. "Florence," an HIV-positive teacher, witnessed an incident while she was getting treatment in the TB ward:

> I remember one lady was reacting to the pills and she throw up again and again. You know, abusive words were herald upon her, (shouting) "hey why do you take a lot of water like that?" Then I started to learn. It was my first time taking those pills at Jubilee hospital. Then, I learned from that, oh I'm not supposed to take a lot of water with my TB pills, I learned from, you know I learned just within that midst of confusion . . . they leave you in ward three, *they just attend people they know are going to adhere* [to TB]. Because you are here for a second time, they say "no you are here for a second time, why?" . . . It is wrong; I mean they should treat people not because of their status, not because of their social status. No, no, no, do you understand what I mean? I was looking at them and I had to fight with other nurse health workers there. Why do you [say that]? Why do you have to shout at that person who has just thrown up? Why don't you tell her that she is not supposed to take too much water with those pills? I only learned when you were shouting at her, you see, and they were coming like they were threatening . . . I did not like that. I'm a person ("Florence").

These observations are somewhat telling. It suggests that the level of care given can be influenced by whether a patient is deemed "good" in terms of their level of adherence or not. The harsh treatment was due to the nurses' exasperation that the patient had apparently failed, for a second time, to adhere to TB medication. Interestingly, the role of status was mentioned with at least two implications.

First, the teacher making these observations suggests that health workers place inadequate focus upon a TB patient's broader social circumstances: for those not adhering, perhaps they have no food, and may use drugs, or drink, or are involved in prostitution. Adherence must be placed in this broader context of social challenges rather than these difficulties being used merely to judge patients and discriminate against them (Chapter 7).

But the second aspect is how a patient's response to the quality of treatment is conditioned by their social status. In this instance, "Florence," a teacher, used her own social status to confront the nurse's harsh treatment of the patient. Unlike the patient treated harshly, "Florence" used her position and social standing to reprimand the nurse's treatment. The role of social class is therefore an additional factor in access and accountability. And this ability to question staff is an issue that will be returned to later in the chapter.

In another instance, a person living with AIDS mentioned how she tested for HIV at Jubilee. But because the nurse knew her, the nurse decided to lie about the test result in order to protect her. The patient was told she was negative. But three months later, she went to another hospital because the symptoms had not gone away. This time she was told her results were positive. So, while the nurse's behavior may be construed as safeguarding the patient, it is nonetheless irresponsible that a health care worker chose to withhold information from a patient, with devastating consequences. Again, it reveals a power dynamic.

A basic level of care and compassion was deemed to be lacking. This was linked to a strong sense of injustice by many, including "T": ". . . some people they are working there but they don't know how to treat somebody who's living with AIDS . . . some people say I rather die at home . . . staying at home than going to Jubilee. Because Jubilee, Jubilee they are going to finish me off. And that is not the right way, because Jubilee is for everyone."

Such concerns were not only expressed by people living with AIDS—they were also shared by some staff. The previous clinical head of Wellness had himself been concerned about the treatment of his patients at the hospital. On one occasion, a patient told him she did not wish to stay in the hospital because she feared for her well-being. This was a feeling also shared by the doctor himself. Patients would often refuse to go to the wards and he would admit them at Wellness because they did not want to go to a medical ward. On this occasion, fearing for the patient's well-being, Dr. Moshabela went himself to fetch the patient in question. He also discovered that a special "code 279" was being used to identify AIDS patients on their files. Often, he claimed, these patients would be placed deliberately in the last cubicle on a ward. The implication was that they would be seen by junior doctors and would have minimal care. As a result of the doctor's complaint, the code was eventually dropped. Another said that at "ward 2 all the nurses, when you go outside, say 'look at this one, she has got AIDS.'" As if to capture the level of discrimination—and its sometimes comical proportions—directed at people living with AIDS, the following account is informative:

"Thando": I was once there to take out a tooth [at Jubilee] you see. Then I explained my situation [HIV status]. You know they called each other . . .

Facilitator: What?

"Thando": They called each other and said come and see

"Wandi": Come and see what?

"Thando": Come and see a HIV person (group laughter). I end up saying to the doctor, "doctor you see, this Aids is giving me a problem," loud,

> in front of everybody. "Make note, the tooth pains, so take it out you see." So that they can feel that I take these things as it is [i.e., the tooth ache was no different from anyone else, HIV positive or not]. This made them ashamed, they just looked at me and said "eish" and look at the others because they called each other, even the other nurses at other rooms they will come and see . . . [just a normal tooth pulling].

An important consideration is whether this general context of discrimination therefore affects use of ARVs. "Rose" recounted a story, again reflecting the role of social status, about a patient using ARVs who was admitted to Ward 2: ". . . one patient was admitted at ward 2 in Jubilee and she was taking the ARVs. But then when she was in the ward they did not give her the ARVs. Her cousin was someone [status]; she came and asked her when she visited 'did they give you your ARVs,' and she said, 'no, since I was admitted in the hospital I did not get my ARVs.' Then she came towards them [the nurses] and explained to them and then they give her the ARVs and she takes it."

Part of the problem concerning attitudes to Wellness patients is also that the nursing staff appears to have little knowledge of ARVs. Some even refused to handle patients on ARVs for fears of toxicity.

A related organizational issue, as suggested by Dr. Cameron, was that there are administrative issues to do with wards passing the buck of burden of care to other wards. This often gave the appearance of negligence. For example, when patients were referred from Jubilee to Wellness, there appeared to be inadequate information given to the patient explaining the transfer:

I think the hospital, when they want to refer someone here they don't tell them . . . they do not say to the people "we are referring you to Wellness clinic, this and this and this is going to happen to you, this is the reason, why we are referring you." They just say go to the Wellness clinic and give him the file . . . they do not explain to them what is going to be . . . done to them, why they are being referred to the Wellness clinic. I think I can say that is one of the ways I can say they are not cooperating very well. Because they are suppose to do as much as they [can] to explain to them when they go . . . or another ward what they are going to do. They need to explain to them you are going to get post counseling so that you can get your results and know your HIV status. (dietician, Wellness)[4]

Upon referral, this is often the first occasion that a patient discovers their HIV status.

In contrast to the main hospital, Wellness itself appears to provide a very different specialization empathetic, and caring environment for people living with AIDS with a team comprising doctors, nurses, dieticians, social workers, and others. But there were similar problems to do with turnover in staff—an issue closely related to administrative issues, as the next section shows—a particularly significant issue for people living with AIDS. The struggle to retain staff and to fill vacancies is an often-cited structural problem confronting South African health services. And these difficulties are disproportionately experienced in more rural areas.[5] This has an impact on both current and future patients' level of care, as expressed by "Thabo":

> If I can give one example; if I start the ARVs I see one doctor, and every time I see that doctor I feel comfortable, you see, yah. But if I have to see different doctors I remember when I had to start ARVs it taken me almost 4 months to take the ARV, you see. Because if today, if I go there I find the other doctor he will say 'no,' you know I was coughing, he said 'you know just go for an X-ray,' I go for an X-ray than I come back you know there is nothing, next month you can start the ARVs. [But] Next month I come I get another doctor he says: 'no, I give this and you start next month.' You see you get different doctors and you don't feel comfortable that time you see.

The turnover in staff can be traumatic for some. Upon finding out about the departure of the first head of Wellness clinic, one of his patients bemoaned: "Yo, I cried when he leave. He told me, he came to me he said you know . . . I'm going to Mpumalanga. I cried you see I really cried. I said to him why, it's a pity" ("Florence"). Many patients were fully aware that new doctors were not specialists in HIV/AIDS. As a result, "T" preferred to make a round-trip to another town, costing R60 because he thought they had more specialist doctors at that facility. And "they know how to handle people who are HIV positive, compared to those at Jubilee." Some Jubilee patients preferred to go directly to the clinic, or, rather than having to go to '"out patients,'" even pay a private doctor rather if they could. "T" described the previous head of Wellness clinic as the "best doctor I ever saw, ever met at the hospital." In his own view, poor administration was responsible for hastening the departure of Dr. Moshabela: ". . . the administrators of the hospital weren't assisting the clinic as good as they could, they were drawing up obstacles."

Wellness was by no means immune to criticism. The problems of waiting, queuing, and getting patient files were identified as "a big problem" at Wellness. Some patients complained that "when the doctors go for lunch they never come back" that day. Another issue was not being given the correct number of pills as "if sometime they don't count pills." They then have to return to the clinic, upon which the patient is told, "no, today it is not your day. We are not going to help you. Wait until 4 p.m., whilst you are the first person there seven o'clock in the morning . . . the problem is with them, they never count the pills." Sometimes pills were damaged, and patients are told not to drink them but then when they go back to clinic, they are told to wait until four o'clock. One respondent said they had experienced negative things at Wellness, such as being late or not getting the right appointment on that day. In addition, some claimed that even here, the receptionists or other staff gossip and do not do so directly to a patient's face but when backs are turned.

Explaining Poor Treatment of Patients

As mentioned earlier, exposing these negative experiences is entirely appropriate in terms of how it may affect patient adherence. But also more generally, if a truly genuine rights-based approach is to be introduced at institutions, one that foregrounds the dignity of the patient and ethical handling by health care workers, a necessary starting position is to explore why these violations take place in the first place.

Health Care Worker Issues

Some issues, such as staffing shortages, have already been mentioned as a critical factor in affecting the quality of care. It is therefore important to remember that health care workers, whilst implicated in violations, may also be victims themselves, along with patients, of what have been described as "highly stressed institutions."[6] In discussions with COSATU representatives, a litany of grievances having to do with forced testing, stigmatization, and breaches of confidentiality directed against employees (not only health but also more generally) became apparent. Quality of care issues would therefore appear enmeshed in broader staff-management relations. These must be fully appreciated and understood if there is to be any improvement. Upon approaching management, a situation of bullying appeared to overshadow any sense of ethical entitlement workers may have: ". . . when you take it further with the management, sometimes they try to convince the person . . . so that he mustn't talk about that [these experiences]. And then they start to threaten him that you know, you are going to lose your job and this and that. That is why I was saying people do not know their rights" (COSATU representative).[7] Work-based HIV initiatives, it was claimed, fell victim to management coercion and desire for controlling the process. What was constructed as a participatory process often entailed co-option of the worker representative by management or board of management, in effect leading to control by the latter. COSATU mentioned the destructive and demoralizing role of performance-related pay and working conditions: "Sometimes we used to blame the nurses or the worker. Whereas there is full stress from the management side you see." This issue is powerfully underpinned in relation to an incident involving a disciplinary hearing of some Jubilee nurses. According to the Legal Resources Centre (LRC), who instigated legal proceedings against the nurses on behalf of the victim's mother, the nurses were implicated in the stillbirth of a baby. LRC had strong evidence to suggest negligent practices led to the stillbirth. But, as suggested above by COSATU, there are also broader structural and institutional issues and policies, which meant that the nurses were also, to some extent, themselves victimized because they had been poorly supervised. Unless we understand grievances on both sides—worker and patient—then it is unlikely that they can be undone by legal interventions alone. It is particularly important to note, as mentioned before and as evident in the 2004 research, that health care workers also have their own considerable constraints and frustrations with hospital management.

The more general shortage of nurses and doctors was highlighted by one doctor as particularly significant. Dr. Cameron suggested that there are too few experienced doctors, and this means less experienced doctors are more likely to give wrong prescriptions, and with too little supervision and too much responsibility.[8] Poor administration, such as salaries not paid on time—in Cameron's case, it was still not properly sorted out after three years—and with basic maintenance not kept up. Some staff also experience HIV-related issues themselves, including forced testing, HIV-related dismissals, breaches of confidentiality, and a general context of limited worker rights and poor working conditions. The coerced testing of workers continues to be related to stigma and negative attitudes to the disease displayed by health care workers.

Another issue raised by some respondents concerns the practice of nepotism at the hospital with management endorsing these practice because: "They don't hire people at Jubilee but put their families in jobs."[9] These types of practices, and concealment of them, and an authoritarian style of management inherited from the Bophuthatswana era, may all be contributory factors for why "the hospital" apparently "has no working relationship with the community."[10]

Access, Quality, and Care

The explanations for why patients are apparently treated as badly as they are in the hospital (rather than Wellness) are indeed complicated. They span structural, historical, and cultural dynamics. But what is critical is to regard such workplace organizational issues as enabling or disabling rights-based approaches. That is, we cannot understand the "quality" of care dimension in the right to health, without contextualizing why bad quality is often more likely. In particular, what assumptions are made about a preexisting conscious rights-holder claimant in rights-based analysis? For example, one explanation for why this is not the case is offered as follows by a patient: "When you go to Jubilee and they do not handle you well, usually we do not talk. We expect that whoever is coming to help us should be the one to talk first. If we can start talking and tell people what we want. At the TB ward, for instance, if they admit you today, they give you treatment but then if there is default they tell you that 'you are wasting our time because we told you to do 1, 2, 3 and you did not do it'"

("Florence"). While the limited capacity of patients to ask questions is perhaps typical the world over, it is particularly constrained in this area. Patients usually do not feel they have legitimacy to influence events, such as a right to ask critical questions in the face of authority. The local political culture and social hierarchy will certainly have a bearing upon this discourse and legitimacy of "answering back." People have rights on paper, often "gold standard" rights but implementing them is another matter altogether. One respondent claimed that the local culture is an issue in that "some cultures don't talk."

Amidst many causal factors, the ghosts of the past historical abuse of people is never far from explaining the present gaps in invoking rights: "Because you know, you cannot give what you don't have. I mean most of us, we have been abused mentally by the apartheid, by our husband, by many, many things you see. So we are, you know, we are withdrawn with shame. [And] some health workers do not have education that is my opinion" ("Florence").

Shame is therefore an important consideration in rights-based approaches. Apartheid health discourse, like its discourse of racial and ethnic separation more generally, was about creating submissive objects rather than rights-bearing subjects (Schneider et al 2007). The role of education—for health care worker and patient alike—was therefore raised. This respondent felt that the role of education to explaining who is more likely to talk back: ". . . you can imagine . . . most of our people are illiterate you understand. *So you will take ARVs not because you want but because you don't understand* . . . really we [those educated] are just fortunate . . . we have been to school or we have Wellness, what about the other greater community? [i.e., surrounding areas] You can imagine in Majanang clinic [rural area not far from Hammanskraal-Temba] there is only one doctor . . . one doctor, she comes on Friday, only this day, and she will never tell you about ARVs" ("Florence"). This raises an important point about the critical role of treatment literacy to empower patients (and, not to forget, the nurses who earlier expressed fears of toxicity of ARVs in handling patients) with a basic level of information. Even if insufficient, it is a necessary starting point and is returned to in the chapter on "alternative medication" and the conclusion. There was consensus in this particular focus group on this issue:

> I agree . . . saying that most of the people are illiterate, they're afraid of asking questions. Myself, when I go to the doctor I rather spend thirty minutes with the doctor, because I know I will question each and every time. And then the patients came to me, I remember last month, they came to me because they were complaining, 'you know you stay for a long time in there.' I told them you know what, this is my life and I have to know more about these things. If I don't ask who then who will help me then? You know? You know people are afraid of asking questions, I don't know why. From my side, I don't want any problems with myself, I ask each and everything that are mainly important questions ("Rose").

As mentioned above, health workers might also lack training or have other grievances. Like their patients, health care workers are also afraid of asserting their rights for fear of repercussion. In response to being asked whether nurses are merely being made scapegoats for more general failings, a key respondent from LRC (the case mentioned earlier in this chapter) replied, "the main problem at Jubilee is bad management . . . People don't realize they have rights and a right to health care, people don't have knowledge and health is not considered an immediate need–therefore people don't come forward [to complain]."[11]

So the link between accountability of management and lack of ability to assert rights is made. In the section on human rights in Chapter 2, if people do not see them as relevant then they are hardly likely to invoke rights. Echoing the work of Høg, a "silence of rights" remains. And, as suggested earlier, people can also be inhibited from complaining for fear of repercussions. For example, one group told how they feared losing their grant, claiming that a local PLWA had lost their grant for failing to adhere to ARVs. So, the basic role of information, through education and training, is identified as an important gap in enabling some basic accountability: "The health workers of Jubilee must have workshops so that they must know how to handle people who are living with HIV and AIDS. They mustn't gossip about them because the others are not strong [to deal with this gossip] like myself" ("T").

Others also had suggestions directed at health workers:

> the health workers . . . have to make it a point that they win the confidence of people so they can [be helped to] cope with the treatment, not just do things rush, rush, rush, going over you know on top of our heads like that you see. If somebody cannot win your confidence, do you understand what it means? It means that there is war between me and you. So most people, most of us, we are not as confident as we are here [clinic support group] today you see, I [would otherwise] just hide about my problem, I will just sit back and I wont tell anybody. I would rather choose to die ("Florence").

Human resource constraints often meant patients felt rushed when at the clinic unless they requested more time: "If you are eager you stay but some people they don't because the way that they [the clinic] tell them you don't have to stay there long . . . maybe you have a question to ask the doctor . . . you don't have a chance, they will tell you don't have side effects, you don't have a problem, they will say take the treatment and . . . go home . . . you see that's where the problem is" ("Sibo"). So the implication is that only those who "stand up" for themselves can tackle such problems. Most do not complain even though they might be experiencing problems. Of course, education and training and the ability to assert oneself individually are important. But so, too, is a more institutionalized response through pressure groups at the grassroots level. An interesting byproduct of the interventions in Hammanskraal has been the emergence—in the absence of the TAC (until 2008) or NAPWA—of an advocacy group formed to contest AIDS-related violations of rights:

> So, as the advocacy committee, we have said . . . Make sure that when someone [i.e., staff] says they are new, look at his or her name tag and make sure that he'll know that he'll write down the name of that person, that sister health worker that he serves in that day. So that when the problem arises he can identify the person who denies you the right. Say 'sister so and so and doctor so and so and so deny me the right the right today checked by the doctor, you know.' That is why we are busy doing that . . . It's gonna work, its gonna give the support group the courage to take to Jubilee to carry to Wellness to get on ARVs. So, then we are going to make a point that, those clerks does not go through their files . . . they must not go through their files. The person who must go through the files is only the doctor not the other health staffs. We insist to form a committee, so that to make people living with HIV and AIDS feel comfortable when they go to Jubilee ("T").

The issue of what creates leverage over accountability will be returned to in the conclusion. But here, it is particularly apt to end this section with reference to the opening quotation at the start of the chapter. It was made by a COSATU representative and appears to capture the significance of institutional governance. This management style deeply constrains the operationalization of a full range of clinic and extra-clinic community-based activities. It is a feature of power that rights—again, if they are to have relevance—should speak to.

Management and Sectoral Collaboration

The Wellness clinic was newly created. As a consequence, it would appear important to have had hospital management support. Yet both successive heads of Wellness described their various frustrations regarding attempts to collaborate with the hospital. The previous head said various ways of putting in mechanisms that required outside collaboration would be proposed but the hospital would apparently feel threatened by this and veto it. As a result, because of apparent failure to cooperate, relationships between the clinic and the district health office, community based organizations, and NGOs were affected, resulting in substantial delays in setting up services.

First, minor, yet essential, hospital functions, such as providing pin codes in order to use the phones as well as more substantial matters, such as provision of transport for patient home visits, were cited as barriers to operating optimally. The latter were identified as increasingly important. Home visits would therefore play a significant role. One female ARV patient, for example, was jokingly told that because she had not been to clinic, the police were looking for her to caution her. This prompted her to cite "problems with money" as the reason for missing her appointment. Humor aside, the role of home visits appears a critical one for many patients (see Chapter 7). But it also indicates, more generally, the subordination of clinicians to budget control of hospital management.

Second, on a more fundamental structural level, the current head of Wellness was, at one stage, the only doctor at the clinic. This put a strain on his ability to do related tasks, such as impairing his time to make visits to the pediatric ward, where referrals to the Wellness clinic could have been made. However, the hospital was apparently not actively seeking to refill vacancies. Accordingly, it became impossible to meet patient targets. So a colleague suggested that he involve an NGO to solve staffing problems. However, the hospital was dead-set against this. It became impossible even to arrange meetings with the managers. They were not happy about it and objected, saying any initiative "must come from us and through us." Whereas this placed the onus upon the clinic head to arrange meetings, it proved near impossible to get any commitment from the hospital to attend. This became apparent when, on several occasions, Tiny Magano, the manager of Jubilee, was approached for a meeting with the Tswelopele project. Each time, however, she was always out of the office. The management at the hospital was described as having a mentality as if: "'We will show you we are so powerful that we will suppress your good intentions: how dare you organize anything without us,' despite me not saying anything is organized, it is merely for you to meet these guys."[12] This is also reflected internally with an apparent schism between management and their own staff.

Fortunately, and illustrative of the influential role of provincial government regarding hospital management, Wellness had sent its obligatory progress report to the provincial health office, who, upon receipt, then inquired as to why the clinic was struggling to meet its targets. It was only after that meeting that the Province agreed that the situation required whatever necessary to help meet targets. But Jubilee management had opposed this. North West is especially concerned about targets and generally has become quite proactive in scaling up its treatment program. They wanted Wellness to initiate fifty patients on treatment per month and to send proper reports or statistics. Again, due to human resource constraints, Wellness could not do so. The provincial level intervention was therefore critical in responding to the clinic's human resource constraints. Currently, through an agreement with an NGO, at least half of the staff is funded through this arrangement, from another doctor, to nurses and even cleaners. While studies indicate the *lack* of the hospital manager's control over administrative decision-making in an overly centralized system—hence with great powers for, often autocratic, provincial decision-makers—within Jubilee, managers appear to exert a lot of power (von Holdt and Murphy 2007). Wellness staff experience frustration, with collaboration initiatives becoming unnecessary power tussles, particularly concerning the management's reluctance to working with "outside" institutions: "And it is why we end up fighting with them [hospital management], I mean, what is the core business of this institution? This clinic is not supposed to be in the hospital, it is supposed to be out there [pointing toward the community] and they just don't understand that. They wanted to have power from that, over that, so they don't like us there. They call us an elite group [laughter]. Because [they think] we want to detail their day-to-day running of things" (social worker).[13] Again, much of the dysfunction is related to what some attribute to a "silo structure of management," reflecting parallel fragmented internal structures, each separately for nurses, doctors, and support workers. Critically, clinicians and nurses do not have a significant role in determining the budget or in monitoring and controlling costs. So, within a disempowering and disjointed system, described for many hospitals, "this generates structural conflict between professional staff and managers . . . clinical heads of department have no idea what their budgets are and costs are not disaggregated within the institution . . . there is no well-structured locus of authority and control within the institution, managers are not accountable for any particular clinical or operational outcome" (von Holdt and Murphy 2007:323). This means that the appearance of authoritarianism may often be related to the essence of a lack of overall structure of accountability at Jubilee, like many other hospitals. But perhaps as damaging as the obstacles to day-to-day operations, there is, however, evidence to suggest that management deliberately creates more insidious barriers. This has had particular effects for any attempts of the ARV clinic to publicize their work and the benefits of ARVs in the community. For example, an arrangement had been made for the head to present the work of Wellness on the local Moretele community radio. Given the level of confusion documented in this study concerning ARVs (see the next two chapters in particular), this appears of particular concern. But the hospital management opposed it. Furthermore, Wellness staff have been prevented from acting on advisory boards for local initiatives (such as the Centre for the Study of AIDS' *Tswelopele* III paralegal project, called "PLACE"). And during the research in *Tswelopele* I, one of the focus groups with nurses, with whom management representatives sat in, clearly felt afraid of saying anything that would be construed as implicating the hospital. So this is illustrative of undermining the clinic's ability to work with other sectors, to name merely a few instances. A number of CBOs also complained that they had difficulties in working with Jubilee.

Another example concerns relations between the district health office and Jubilee, often described as poor. As if to illustrate the poor communication, a gate between the two adjacent work places had apparently been closed. Although it was claimed this was for security reasons, and especially for theft of property, it is hard to perceive it as other than poor relations. More recently, district health has been involved in working with defaulting patients. A list of such patients had been presented to the district health by Wellness regarding patients who had abandoned treatment (measured by period of absence). District health claimed it was working well because it was integrated with program within Jubilee, which illustrates that these issues can be overcome with will.

Another example was cited by a social worker who had an offer from Soul City to do training with the clinic's support group. Management reiterated its stance that if people are coming from outside, they must first be given an invitation. As a result, attempts were made to get hold of the general manager to issue invitations but it was impossible to get an appointment to do so. The upshot was that, "people are not getting information, information that is going to make them better people, and make them better empowered" (unnamed respondent). Furthermore, regarding staffing, the clinic was supposed to get its own principal pharmacist, an issue mentioned in the context of drug shortages, when adults were given pediatric syrup due to the shortage of one particular drug. And in another case, treatment was only available for one week. The social worker raised concerns that this did not encourage adherence because patients may not have money to come back after only one week. So, whereas the clinic and the national treatment program more generally may preach adherence, supply factors may undermine this. Indeed, one respondent spoke of being told to come back the next day for treatment, which she regarded as effecting her ability to adhere, not least due to the extra transport costs. These broader collaboration issues were illustrated, again, in efforts to get a pharmacist: "Hospital management kidnapped the whole situation and did not want to offer the post as the hospital already had one . . . I feel that if we had one person that was managing this at all times you know she'll be able to advocate for what is correct . . . what drugs are running short, what can I do to assist you."[14] To this date, the clinic still does not have its own pharmacist.

What, therefore, is underpinning management's hostility and suspicion? On one level, the phrase "elite" clinic does appear to express resentment and rivalries between the clinic and older and more established sections. Perhaps management perceives the clinic to be receiving funds disproportionate to their own. Or, perhaps it is the "special" nature of AIDS that creates divisions. On a deeper level, it was suggested by some respondents that Jubilee behaves in such a fashion because they are fearful that collaborative working relationships might mean some of their working practices are exposed to scrutiny. There may be corrupt practices occurring and management would like to leave these unexposed. One anonymous respondent highlighted the lack of transparency and lack of consultation associated with a culture of institutional secrecy. I was told, "they [the hospital] don't like to transform."

The differences between the clinic and Jubilee were duly noted by respondents in the focus groups, that is, those receiving care and therefore directly affected by lack of collaboration. One example given concerns the celebration of World AIDS Day at Jubilee, which apparently did not have any specific involvement of people living with AIDS, described by one as a disgrace. The gap between Jubilee and Wellness was described as, "it's like two hospitals in one ground." Another respondent cited the role of management in particular "as if they are not working for the same Department of Health. That there is a problem with the people. They are meant to be a team." What, then, about broader governance of local AIDS initiatives?

Local AIDS Council

The apparent difficulties of intersectoral collaboration between Jubilee and the broader community would appear to make the Local AIDS Council's role in mobilizing different stakeholders even more important. The first research project period uncovered profound disappointments with the Local Aids Council (LAC). A series of well placed local NGOs, community organizations, and Tshwane municipality informants indicated that the LAC was not delivering on its mandate. Although it was established in 2000, it had not become active until 2004. Then, in the unlikely event of a CBO or NGO being awarded funding, the LAC apparently sought to dictate what should be done with the funding. This intervention and also the apparent lack of commitment to non-LAC initiatives appeared to be related to the politicized nature of the LAC and its inability to differentiate between "politics and the disease" ("Jacob"). In other words, politicians, i.e., councillors, including its then chair, were capturing the LAC for partisan purposes. An important local traditional leader, Chief Nawa, identified the LAC as part of the municipal structure with whom he and other traditional leaders felt their power base was being challenged. These differences are hardly conducive to intersectoral collaboration via the LAC. When the LAC was approached for comment, at that time, the (since ex-) chair suggested that these views were only a misperception that they were not responding, when in fact LAC engages with local stakeholders. She claimed that the problem lay with local people who needed to take ownership. Furthermore, by 2007, the LAC's Area coordinator also suggested that while it was very keen to forge partnerships, problems existed with the potential collaborating organizations. He claimed this reflected an apparent "trade-off" of such organizations being 60 percent commitment against 40 percent of those uncommitted. He gave an example of linking a disadvantaged community and a woman with terminally ill clients not served by any clinic with the hospital board in order to resolve the matter by providing a mobile clinic. But another source claimed that political leaders, for example, had commandeered positions at the LAC and demanded that the area coordinator drive them to meetings in Mmabatho and elsewhere. Most damaging of all were critical comments directed at the LAC concerning lack of transparency in finances. One respondent (anonymous) revealed how, at one meeting, the LAC budget statement given was identical to that of the preceding year. In other words, there appears to be lack of accountability regarding the funding situation of the LAC, further worsening the already precarious reputation of the LAC.

The negative comments directed at the LAC were not confined to civil society. To illustrate how the LAC is apparently more preoccupied with spending money on themselves and functions rather than delivering any programs, a Moretele Municipality employee (KI 18) commented that "they (LAC) only ring me when they have a function." That such poorly functioning structures are not held accountable contributes to patchy local intersectoral collaboration. These have profound consequences for delivery of ARV and associated health services.

The issues raised in this chapter provide an overview of institutional issues in quality of care. As such, they throw down a number of challenges to ARV use and rights-based approaches. These issues may also be highly significant in relation to feeding into broader and fiercely contested public claims and counterclaims made about ARVs impact upon individuals. It is therefore important to turn now to assessing what people living with AIDS think of ARV treatment, both prior to and following their own initiation onto treatment.

CHAPTER 5

Social Acceptability

Stigma, Social Attitudes, and the ARV Information Gap

Previous chapters have indicated some of the institutional hurdles people living with AIDS need to negotiate if they are to access ARVs. But long before they get to the clinic and begin the ARV enrolment process, a significant hurdle concerns the way in which ARVs are commonly perceived. Contrary to the generally accepted medical rationale that ARVs can prolong life, a quotation by "Thandi" in the Introduction appears to fly in the face of the evidence. Some are depicting ARVs as generating fear rather than vanquishing it. Since the *Tswelopele* project at the Centre for the Study of AIDS commenced in 2004, many respondents have observed that stigma associated with AIDS is lessening over time. But stigma's continuing role in accessing treatment remains complex and resilient. Explaining where the fear associated with ARVs comes from calls for unpacking it at different levels. How social attitudes are vested in perceptions of ARVs is one critical dimension. Another concerns the role of treatment education and information and whether this is adequately provided in order to challenge some of the fears. Above all, if the prevailing climate is one of fear, the role of national leaders would appear crucial in seeking to address such concerns. Whether this alone can allay personal denial is also debatable. This chapter explores these issues.

Attitudes Before and After Accessing ARVs

Prior to accessing treatment at the clinic, it is reasonable to suggest that ARVs are not regarded in a positive light within this community. On the one hand, people in the community still encounter a lot of AIDS-related death and illness. People living with AIDS explained that they were seeing people getting access to treatment but that they were still dying. It was common to regard ARVs themselves as responsible. Of course, there is a need to untangle the factors involved in mortality as distinct from the role of treatment *per se*. But the point remains that ARVs are associated with death and desperation in that people take ARVs as a last resort when they are already in an advanced stage of illness. One current patient at the Wellness clinic relayed that she had been "very scared when people they talked about ARVs" because she thought that people only take them when they are already dying.[1] People living with AIDS talked about people they knew who were adamant they would not take ARVs because they do not help and actually kill. This appears to reflect, as recounted by the respondents themselves, a fundamental problem in that people are going to access ARVs very late, when they are already seen as ill, even terminal. Many recounted how they only found out about ARVs when they were ill and had been tested and introduced to the Wellness program. This represents something of a catch-22: ARVs remain associated with death but people only hear about them when they have already approached the clinic, usually after having fallen ill.

Some of the more commonly cited negative attitudes to ARVs involve side effects and associated rumors: ". . . some say you will go mad, get nightmares . . ." ("Rose"). ARVs are associated with "problems" and this is what people hear about. Others indicated their fear at being told by health care workers that the ARVs would be for life, "then I ask myself this is for life and what happens if I miss the time [when I should take pills]?" ("Sibo"). One respondent said that he, like others, heard much about ARVs that they did not understand and were attempting to sift through the rumors to hear from those on treatment themselves. But uncertainties circulate within this community, culminating for one patient, as seen earlier, in his association of ARVs with being a "gamble." Other related factors cited by respondents include anxieties related to the requirement they heard about regarding adherence. This implied, for them, that friends or family also need to be involved: "You know, if you hear about something you don't know about, there are so many thing that come to your mind. The first time I heard about ARVs was 'come with your buddies.' I began asking myself many questions, why did they want my buddies?" ("Rose"). Another was scared to access ARVs because she was told her parents had to accompany her to the clinic. Whilst this may or may not be associated with a requirement to disclose (see Chapter 7), it appears to heighten anxiety for some. Undoubtedly, other factors are also interlinked into generating fears. The first two successive heads of Wellness clinic reiterated the role of the emotional baggage patients come with prior to commencing treatment. The head at the time of writing, Dr. Mathibedi, explained that when patients are about to start treatment, the majority does so with reservations. In particular, the most common questions concern the toxicity of ARVs and especially whether they work: "And when you interrogate them as to why and then you realize that they have fears. Either they know someone who died or someone suffering side effects. They start treatment with reservations and to say that it is toxic is quite common" (Dr. Mathibedi).[2] Such uncertainties were also mentioned by the first head of Wellness, Dr. Moshabela.[3] He identified a tendency for patients to mention side effects and also to place emphasis upon toxicity rather than any of the benefits of ARVs. The dietician at Wellness also confirmed these perceptions that ARVs "are dangerous or they are toxic" and reflect inadequate information.[4] To gauge such attitudes toward treatment, a questionnaire was given to members of the Wellness support group. It revealed that of the thirteen members responding to the question of whether they perceived ARVs as positive or negative: 76 percent (ten) said positive; 7.7 percent (one) said negative; 7.7 percent (one) said both positive and negative; and 7.7 percent (one) was positive but fearful of toxicity. Although a small sample, and also bearing in mind the presence of the clinic social worker, which may have prompted some responses, what is interesting to note is the difference in attitude amongst respondents. Whereas those who had commenced treatment responded to the question "positively," those not on treatment replied negatively. This difference most likely reflects the benefits—as stated on numerous occasions more generally by the Treatment Action Campaign, for example—of being introduced to treatment information and getting additional information through membership of a treatment support group. Conversely, those not on treatments included the one "negative" person and also the person scared about toxicity. This appears to confirm a more general trend constituting an information gap. To illustrate the lack of information on ARVs, this uncertainty also pertained to health workers. One patient, "Florence," said she had been asked by her clinic to teach the staff about ARVs. Again, although there may be reservations about this being a very small "captured" sample, it nonetheless reveals that those citing toxicity fears and negative attitudes were more likely *not* to be on treatment. In other words, this mirrors the focus group discussions wherein both people living with AIDS on treatment discussed their fears and anxieties *prior* to commencing treatment, for reasons stated. Furthermore, the non-PLWA "control" group also voiced the generalized fears rooted in community perceptions of ARVs.

The concerns mentioned here serve to highlight a more general issue: ARVs have an image problem and are being associated with negative attributes prior to treatment. Ideas are placed into a person's mind before they even commence treatment. If the loss of life is not already devastating enough, these deaths continue to reinforce whatever negative perceptions some people living with AIDS and the community may harbor concerning ARVs. Before looking at some additional factors shaping perceptions—and this is particularly significant because it is likely to act as a source of aggravation of broader adherence problems, all of which affect "access"—the question of whether such perceptions change following commencement of treatment will be addressed.

Attitudes After Treatment: What Happens to Stigma?

> Yah! That is why people were scared to go fetch treatment from Jubilee for instance because of this stigma. They were scared that some would look at them and say that their lives are over . . .
>
> —"Thandi"

As suggested, paradoxically, life-giving treatment remains associated with "lives that are over," as one PLWA pointed out in the quotation above. Having noted the links between perceptions of ARVs and illness and death, one particular question raised is therefore why this association is not eroding a connection with death. After all, this positive association has been a powerful claim of treatment activists (Heywood n.d.). The majority of respondents, for example, did note how they felt strong and healthy after side effects had been controlled. The physical benefits were substantial, so much so that one respondent, "Florence," the teacher, had returned to working life at her school following commencement of ARVs. But even in this positive case, "Florence" still encountered stigmatization by the principal, who refused to shake her hand when she returned to work due, she says, to her HIV positive status.

In an earlier piece of work in Hammanskraal, the construction of stigma was explored (Zuberi et al 2004). Drawing upon the framework created by Link and Phelan (2001), and adding additional components particularly relevant in the context of AIDS, stigma was revealed as a multifaceted, complex social process. Far from social science jargon, the benefit in this approach is to see stigma as a product of a number of components. These include physical appearance, labeling of differences, fears of contagion, and then additional issues identified in the Tswelopele project context of the epidemic, such as promiscuity, bewitching, gendering, and, especially, community-based gossiping. Even now, in the treatment era, a person is still being labeled negatively as "HIV-positive": "People at first, when you have HIV and now you have flu, they would say that, 'no, you are HIV positive.' Flu is one of the symptoms of HIV . . . they would look at you, [even] if you[r] feet are giving you a problem and then say it's HIV, as if everything is HIV!" (unnamed respondent). The scenario is a sequence commonly recited that includes selection of negative connotations between AIDS and physical appearance and fear of contagion. But, as suggested, stigma remains more than these attributes alone. One fundamental indicator of decreasing stigma in the treatment era would be, for example, whether patients are more likely to disclose their HIV positive status to their partner. With all hope of treatment eroding stigma, "Rose," however, suggested: "One other thing that makes people not disclose their status to their partners is that some know that thing [ARVs] is for life. Now what if I tell my partner that I have a big ache, my body is painful and I decided to buy this treatment and after a month everything is going to be okay? [S]He knows that I have to hide myself because my partner is going to realize that this guy last month was drinking this and [s]he is drinking this [i.e taking ARV medication] again, what is going on?" Echoing that dimension of stigmatization closely associated with alleged promiscuity, for some couples, ARVs can therefore signify infidelity. These connotations are not eroded through treatment—on the contrary, they might even be exacerbated. Similarly, when asked if they could take their treatment openly in front of family, in reply, most respondents at best remained in awkward silence. At worst, some claimed they were not free to openly take treatment: "Ha . . . most of the people . . . they take the ARVs and their family doesn't know about their status. When comes the time that he is supposed to take his or her medication, he hide his or herself so the family mustn't see him drinking the medication. The people . . . *they are not free, they are not free.* That is why when some people they say, even if my CD4 account can be zero, I won't take ARVs" ("T").[5] This reflects that some people living with AIDS are fearful of being exposed as being HIV-positive. The role of treatment in this is apparent. One respondent described how people at home, upon seeing so many tablets, would start to comment about this. They would ask, "Why are you taking so many tablets. What is wrong with you and all the things like that and there is nothing you can do." In one group, "Rose" mentioned her neighbor, who goes to the clinic and gets ARVs for a month at a time but who would put them inside the cupboard and "doesn't want to drink them." Another commented: "There are those who take the treatment and throw it away immediately after collecting it. There are some who take it [from the clinic] and put it in the cupboard. Come the day when he passed away you get all the containers still sealed [i.e., unused]." This then prompted one respondent to describe the burial of her neighbor that had happened in the week before the group discussion. Following the funeral, a cupboard of sealed tablets was discovered. The neighbor had apparently "given up caring." Some patients described coping mechanisms for their own treatment use. This was described as "faking" treatment, in other words, concealing the real treatment by using a false label: "Me, what I do is, when I go home I have a container which I got from the chemist. So I pour my pills into this container. People know how ARVs look like but then when they are in this container they are all mixed together so no one will know anything" ("Nonni"). "Florence" mentioned how returning to work meant that she had to take treatment during the day. Although she had been vocal about her status to her colleagues, she found it frustrating when having to take pills in the common room with so many people inquiring what the medication was for. There appeared to be big differences between the focus groups concerning levels of disclosure and freedom to take medication. An important correlation—as evident in more general understating of treatment behavior—lies in the greater the support received, the more openness ensues. Notably, one group in particular seemed to have the highest level of support and far less need to conceal treatment. They spoke of the supportive role of friends and family in reminding them to take treatment and/or setting alarms on mobile phones.

This notion of hiding or concealing treatment was particularly disturbing because it inevitably creates stress, especially of being "found out." The implication is that adherence is made much harder to cope with. When one group was asked whether they knew of people in this category, the same female respondent in the quote concerning her neighbor hiding medication talked about her own brother who, though seriously ill, refuses to go to the Wellness clinic: "I know them; one of them is my brother. He is having a big problem. He is even afraid to go to the hospital. He is using the traditional healer's medication. I even spoke to him on Saturday about ARVs and he promised that he will go to the Wellness [clinic] on Tuesday." There seemed to be two major strands to this explanation. One consisted of the fear of telling his partner, and that can be part of the guilt and denial associated with AIDS. But there was also an association with alternative beliefs. The treatment in question was that encouraged by the Church of Zion (ZCC) referred to as "strong coffee," that is, coffee made from "holy water." The role of alternative and traditional medication is so significant that it receives its own chapter (see Chapter 6). In the case of the brother not wanting to access ARV treatment, it appeared to be less about concerns about the side effects of ARVs—because it was claimed by the sister that "he doesn't know about ARVs"—than about his lack of acceptance of the disease and failure to disclose it to his girlfriend. This denial or hiding of status was also an issue for another woman because, she claimed, her child's father "is hiding his status." It appears to be deeply embedded in personal denial. The patient herself suggested that treatment alone cannot shift this attitude. Asked whether her brother could conceal taking the treatment from the girlfriend, she replied, "ARVs are different from the other medication. Sometimes you drink it as twenty-five pills then his girlfriend is going to ask him why he drinks so many pills. It is better that he tells her or go with her to the clinic and do some tests." Again, the pills themselves signify disease and indicate shame or infidelity. Treatment has become a signifier and in itself is associated in the minds of some people living with AIDS with (involuntary) disclosure. This was described by "T": "Because ARVs makes the community aware that you are HIV positive. The ARVs is one of the major things that causes that stigmatization and then people are not free. And basically this discrimination is caused by ARVs, because most of the people they know that somebody drinking ARVs, it means that that person is HIV positive . . . If you are not brave enough you can't stand this." Whether this can be blamed on the ARVs is, however, an important issue. The shame apparently visited upon families by AIDS, as identified in the 2004 research, was still connected to individual denial and family denial. Many respondents explained this persisted because of the role of ignorance. But upon more recent reflection, perhaps what they really mean is that the issues around stigma and discrimination and common perceptions of the illness were manifesting themselves as denial. Fears and anxieties surrounding AIDS were an important blockage to "access," not access to ARVs *per se*. Confusion was therefore related to those considered in denial. One respondent replied that it has nothing to do with the medication but, rather, denial. She cited her cousin's parents who were hiding their symptoms and status. This pattern of people "hiding away," in other words, in denial about their status, was commonly cited and described as "too many" that are doing it (i.e., "hiding"). First, in some quarters, stigma was regarded as preventing people from accessing treatment from Wellness because as soon as they are seen at the clinic, they are identified as someone with HIV/AIDS. This respondent, a Local AIDS Council co-coordinator, also mentioned breach or fear of breach of confidentiality as an inhibiting factor for many people living with AIDS to approach the clinic. "T" suggested that "many" people were throwing away ARVs for two key reasons: first, they think ARVs are not good for them and will worsen their condition, and second, this stigma means that they do not want people to realize they are on ARVs because it is " . . . medication drunk by people with AIDS." This aspect of denial was most strongly evoked by "Rose," who claimed that, "even if there is going to be a cure; people are still going to continue dying. Those who are in denial, they deny but come the next hour, that same person [belatedly] says 'could you please take me to the clinic, I want to get ARVs. I have heard that ARVs could help.'" The following exchange illustrates this dynamic concerning stigma as discouraging access:

Facilitator: "Do you think there are many people who are not going to the clinic?

"R*ose" and "Nonni"(together):* yah!

"Rose": Most of the people, they are not going to the clinic.

Facilitator: Why do you think they are not going to the clinic?

"Nonni": I think that they are afraid of being stigmatized. They are afraid of being labeled.

The fear of stigma and the denial of status therefore set back access to treatment because it encourages late presentation at the clinic: "You test HIV positive and then you sit down and say that you are not fighting but then the HIV is still going on. Later, you now go to fetch the treatment and now you want to start with the ARVs but then this is not where you should start at [i.e., this is at a very late stage]. When you realize that you are HIV positive you should start with the treatment because your age is not waiting for you and rather than going for treatment you have lost your strength so you should not take this risk" ("Sibo").

So, although the medication is available, doctors must understand the persistence of associated stigmatization that acts as a deterrent for people living with AIDS to seek ARVs. It was apparent in group discussions that many participants, for example, had not disclosed their status beyond the support group. Many felt awkward about disclosure. In one case, even having a friend from the support group was problematic. If they encountered this person whilst walking along the road with parents or relatives and the parents asked where they had met this new friend, inevitably, if they replied the support group, then this implied disclosure of status. Another woman, "Nonni," made an appeal to the support group not to point her out to others if they saw her in the street: "People, I am kindly asking everyone who is here not to tell your friends about me when you see me walking down the street. If you say to your friend that this one is like me I will discipline you in front of your friends."

Those working with HIV-related organizations are labeled "positive." According to Minkie, the leader of a home-based care organization, the role of gossip remains prominent, implicating her work: "They just want to stay [with]in the fence [of their house] and point . . . until they have a patient in their house."[6] So, to overcome this stigma requires substantial social support and a tough personality. Some therefore expressed defiance, stating "I will get the treatment but those who are suffering are those who worry themselves. I go to Jubilee to get my treatment and I do not care." But examples of stigma were also given by others beyond the people living with AIDS respondents. Indeed, outside of support groups, lack of support was evident. The COSATU representatives, for example, had been involved in a case of a hospital employee (at another hospital) who had been prevented from working in the kitchen due to sores on her arms. Rather than providing gloves and training, the woman, they claimed, had been stigmatized to a point whereby stress and anxiety had contributed to her illness and death.

In another area, *Stinkwater*, where most people on ARV treatment obtain this from Jubilee, "Gwen," a middle-aged woman, described the consequences of disclosing her status. In 2002, she was diagnosed HIV-positive. She disclosed her status to her church and sought spiritual healing. Instead of supporting her, the church expelled her. In addition, her husband left her, apparently due to her status. She also experienced intense gossiping by her neighbors. This, she suggested, reflected that "even in the streets people don't like me due to the status." That this stigma apparently persists, following this person's commencement on ARVs, again underscores the complexity of stigma. To illustrate this, Gwen recalled that during disputes with neighbors, it was not uncommon for them to retort, "Go and take your ARVs." Again, given there may well be many other different reasons for the manifestation of stigma directed at this specific woman, that such comments are made nonetheless illustrates the transfer of stigma onto treatment itself.

Whilst stigma comes out as hugely significant in the focus groups, it is surprisingly absent from the questionnaire. In fact, only two respondents mention stigma and/or lack of support as factors affecting access and adherence. But then, 20 percent of respondents in the category of groups facing "hardest" access do identify those "in denial" or "not knowing their status," which could be an indication of the role of stigma in determining access for some. Furthermore, an additional respondent suggested the "fear of ARV," again possibly linking this itself to stigma (which came out strongly in focus groups). This might also indicate that these respondents have support mechanisms (although one clearly does not) and they have gone through stigmatization processes. Additionally, the role of disclosure in access to treatment has not been identified in the questionnaire but came out strongly in focus groups regarding treatment preparation (see Chapter 7). Thus, it could be that the support these respondents get, having disclosed to someone (at the very least to the support group), reduced stigma. People living with AIDS on treatment, and particularly susceptible to stigma, perhaps not in a support group, may not be reflected in the questionnaire sample.

Given this palpable level of anxiety surrounding ARVs, it would appear important to look at the role of public and political messages about ARVs. But do these address such fears and make medication more socially acceptable?

Information and Leadership

Accessing treatment appears to encompass a range of complex issues, integral to which is the the role of local attitudes toward, and perceptions of, ARVs. A vital component is the role of information in enabling informed choices. The majority of respondents in the questionnaire (over 90 percent) gave solid, knowledge-based answers addressing the importance of time management, CD4 counts, and personal motivations and commitments to treatment, and recited its benefits. This might be explained by the presence of the clinic social worker who encourages such awareness. But it nonetheless does reveal a good fundamental understanding of significant factors in adherence and access to treatment. This suggests, therefore, that those "prepared" for treatment, and members of support groups where these issues are discussed in this area, have been exposed to a significant degree of information. But it is important to remember that these are people who have initiated treatment. And many of them continue to experience sociocultural barriers to access (as the next two chapters explore). There are as many, if not more, who would qualify in terms of clinical eligibility but continue not to approach the clinic. The question of whether ARVs are "known" to the community was therefore introduced to all groups. The responses were almost universal, indicating a severe information vacuum encountered by the community in general. Some general information informing people that ARVs are available was provided through television and radio. There appears to be a major information divide between those accessing ARVs and those not accessing them. In other words, for the community at large, "they don't know about ARVs, if you go ask them even the community around, ask them about ARVs, they don't know. Only people who go to Wellness clinic are the ones that know about ARVs" ("Florence"). In terms of more nuanced information and details about the benefits of ARVs, the following views were shared:

> At the present moment, the radio will talk about ARVs saying there is roll-out . . . But awareness of educating people about ARVs, there is nothing. I have not heard one radio or one community radio or TV. On TV they talk about ARVs, you have to take ARVs on time, but they don't tell people about the side effects and what can the ARVs cost you when you are not taking it properly, or, when you mix it with other things. It is only those who are on ARVs, they know that if you are on ARVs you must not drink, you must not smoke; you must not mix with other tablets, with other medications. ("T")

With high levels of illiteracy and limited access to newspapers, one obvious avenue for getting information on ARVs should be the local Moretele community radio. But a radio presenter with a weekly slot on AIDS-related issues said that it was instead currently used to address "alternative medications." Part of the explanation given was that the local hospital had not given permission for the [previous] head of the clinic to promote ARVs on the radio (see Chapter 4 on governance and sectoral collaboration). But on the broadcaster's side, with income generation deemed critical for survival, airtime was being bought through sponsorship and advertisements by those promoting herbal remedies, immune boosters, and other products.

Specific actors—such as government—were identified as responsible for this situation: "People like the Wellness or the government who are issuing ARVs to us, they don't give enough information, you see. The information is just lean"

("Thando"). A particularly significant dimension was leaders who attached negative attributes to ARVs:

> . . . our leaders should nt say negative things about ARVs. People were going to go for ARVs freely without any fear. Some would go to take ARVs, but they could fear that the ARVs on other hand is going to be fire because they have heard that our leader have said that in public . . . So people who wanted to take ARVs, he mustn't be frightened, or made afraid. He [government] was supposed to make them to be free to go to and take ARVs. Because most of the people they said, "I rather die instead of taking ARVs, because I see most of the people who are taking ARVs, are becoming . . . more weak and weaker." ("T")

Yet more respondents observed, " . . . we heard many things about ARVs, we never understand, but are adding the information now [i.e., once actually on it]" ("Thando"). And how, they suggested, beyond Wellness information, there was limited access because "no [one] beyond Wellness clinic are talking about them, the general clinics they don't talk about them" ("Florence"). Other groups expressed similar views. She also indicated the role of an "information gap" in suggesting, "because they did not go into publicity to explain about ARVs. You just have to go to the hospital to know about ARVs." In addition, others cited the fact that there were still few role models in terms of public disclosure: "I think we can disclose to the radios, TVs and some newspapers. If I can say that I'm so and so staying at . . . I started experiencing my HIV/AIDS, maybe I'm twelve years [with] HIV. I'm living with AIDS and I am living on ARVs and they help me so much. I think then that people will change some life styles and start to take some medication" ("Rose"). The scant access to information in surrounding rural areas was considered a particular disadvantage, with suggestions that this is "why the person is weak that he can not take the ARVs, you see. It is because of the information that we get" ("Thando"). Another dimension to the paucity of information was that it served to encourage speculation about ARVs. One respondent expressed concern at what they felt was perhaps their government deliberately hiding information from them. ARVs were considered by some as a mixed blessing—benefiting many but at the same time not always good for people. The absence of adequate information—a vacuum, in effect—appeared to fuel suspicion about ARVs: "You drink ARVs today, tomorrow you die, why? There is a question why. You don't drink ARVs, you drink ARVs today, tomorrow you leave them, some people they don't die they just stay like that [there is] still a question why?"("Thando"). There were anxieties, therefore, even for those on treatment. Much remained unclear for people living with AIDS, with the above comments attributed to someone actually on treatment. The two men raising these issues in this discussion in the group saw themselves as benefiting from ARVs but still felt that, more generally, skepticism was rooted in the community because of lack of information. Some clearly felt they were not being told about both the advantages and disadvantages *before* taking ARVs. Again, the role of government was identified in this: "Even the government must involve itself in giving people the ARVs. But because of not wanting to they will say instead 'we are taking you into the program.' But they won't tell you that the ARVs sometimes can destroy you . . . if you are being fair to people . . . it will say it is my [i.e., informed] choice . . . To me I find they are hiding something . . . they will tell you only the ARVs can do it" ("Thando"). The lack of adequate information—or mixed messages—therefore related to lack of ability to make informed choices one way or another. In other words, not enough information was given to combat adverse perceptions of ARVs but, similarly, a full picture was not given about ARVs as not likely to benefit *all* patients. Even at the clinic level, there were conflicting opinions. For example, some people living with AIDS were unclear about the role of alternative medication, such as *Immunodu*. There appeared to be conflicting information at the clinic level as to whether this should be mixed with ARVs or not: "Yah, within the clinic you see, then you ask yourself: What is the relevant information? You see. And where do I get the relevant information? You see. And then if you ask they will say you are asking too much, you see. You are asking too much, you see, you seem to know too much" (unidentified male). More generally, there appears to be very little debate. The lack of debate was also linked to the wider picture of treatment being a heavily politicized issue. Some health care and social workers also alluded to the role of politics: ". . . the whole ARV thing, I think it had too much controversy around it and that is actually affecting the delivery of services . . . it is too political . . ." (social worker).[7] This had apparently affected preparations at the hospital. Another employee, in district health, also regarded the whole issue as too politicized. But, interestingly, he juxtaposed the minister of health as wishing to introduce a more nuanced side to the debate, with nutrition as the vehicle to discuss complexity of treatment to community members often "impatient" to get ARVs without the necessary education. Another described the minister of health's approach as "she is trying," as well meaning, and as reflecting a collective level of desperation. Whatever the political affiliation of these respondents is, and this is unclear, it does show that the elite discourse resonates at a local level. Issues such as the minister of health's promotion of beetroot and garlic were clearly mentioned by the local radio and, as an earlier section indicated, is usually given credence to. But in the same breath that respondents can regard the fallibility of individuals and individual behavior as largely responsible for the problem in the first place, they can also invoke rights as integral to responses. But these responses are therefore often ambiguous. A respondent can appear to be broadly supportive of the minister of health's philosophy but then criticize government for not doing enough to regulate training and initiation into being a *Sangoma*. There appears to be competing interpretations of citizenship, science, and ARVs, and different conceptions of the role of patients as active actors in their own right, or passive recipients requiring protection, because they cannot look after themselves. This has major implications for the quality of service being provided and, moreover, the ability to hold providers accountable. This chapter has indicated, however, that a range of sociocultural obstacles in accessing treatment exists over and beyond leaders. These certainly challenge the assumptions that have been made about treatment and the hope that it would erode stigma and discrimination easily.

One particular obstacle discussed across all focus groups, and that featured prominently during interviews, concerns the strong undertone of traditional and alternative medication. This seems to reflect a particular area of dereliction of duty on behalf of government. But it is clearly one that should not overshadow how popular impulses exist toward the embrace of traditional and alternative medication.

CHAPTER 6

Cultural Beliefs and Business in an Era of ARVs

> The problem is that of belief. There are those who believe that when you go to the traditional doctors you will get help though there is no cure about HIV/AIDS. Those who believe that when you go to the traditional healers you are going to be healed
>
> —"Florence"

Such comments, as above, could have been attributed to a person living with AIDS in a semi-urban settlement in just about any country in sub-Saharan Africa. Consulting traditional and alternative practitioners is, of course, also a rapidly growing business in many countries in the so-called West and has been commonplace for centuries in Southeast Asia. Whether the rapidly booming popularity of alternative practices evident now in the United Kingdom, or the millennia old practice of consulting traditional healers in China, or *Saami* shaman in Norway, patients have diverse perceptions of illness and therefore its treatment. But in the Southern African region, dealing with its acute predicament as the epicenter of the global epidemic, traditional and alternative perceptions have a particularly significant role in the context of HIV/AIDS interventions and, specifically, in this chapter, ARV programs. These perceptions do not reflect merely a fringe section of society but in fact comprise the mainstream itself in South Africa.

During the quite sensational proceedings of the court case dealing with rape allegations against Jacob Zuma (Chapter 1), amidst all the other more controversial issues that swirled around the case and received attention, different readings of AIDS treatment also surfaced in the national consciousness. Zuma encouraged the HIV-positive complainant to use traditional herbal medication to treat her condition. That there appear to be such different readings of, or at least, in Zuma's case, ones he claims are complimentary to, established scientific truths and evidence-based understandings about HIV/AIDS, goes to the core of the poor responses in tackling the epidemic. Certainly, this can be manifested as poor leadership. And we have seen that political elites have had a lot to say about the science of AIDS and traditional/alternative medication within the context of broader interpretations of the epidemic. But it should appear important to pose the following question: have these elite representations made by the obvious political players—especially the then minister of health and Mbeki—closed down more serious attempts to discuss traditional and alternative treatments as something other than merely used to discredit ARVs? Zuma, for example, contrary to partial media depictions of his testimony concerning HIV transmission during the rape case, is not regarded as an AIDS denialist. Yet, he appears to see a role for the use of traditional medication *and* ARVs. Over and beyond elite political figures, what, therefore, is the grassroots perception of traditional and alternative medication amongst those taking ARVs?

The chapter seeks to provide some explanations of why traditional medication should be so appealing in the context of the AIDS treatment era. There is an emerging, but sadly belated, awareness of the significance of cultural perceptions of health and illness in designing and implementing AIDS-related health interventions. This was learned the hard way through failure of prevention programs. But it is also something still being learned in the context of ARV programs. Even when not overlain by heated political contest, the terrain of belief and health interventions is indeed a very complicated one. What follows in this chapter is therefore an account intended to give a snapshot of a particular community attempting to come to terms with the advent of the ARV era at a particular moment. In this account, attention is given to the key participants—especially people living with AIDS themselves—within the everyday spaces where perceptions of disease and medication are (re)produced in a community. Beyond the fiercely contested claims and counterclaims about medication and the science of AIDS, if we are serious about following human rights considerations in ARV treatment, however, an important dimension is that health services should strive not only to be socially acceptable and of sufficient quality but also *culturally acceptable* to users (Toebes 2001). Can we say this about ARV programs with any certainty?

Fields of Treatment

Spending time in Hammanskraal/Temba quickly reveals that conventional AIDS treatment—ARVs—have to compete with a parallel universe of treatment options, particularly those deemed "traditional" and "alternative." The most popular healers do not need to advertise, as word of mouth makes reputations. Others may daub their trade as "herbalist" in large whitewashed letters adorning the sides of shacks. Many are now also setting up within shopping malls, be they in the inner-city areas of Johannesburg, or more affluent ones such as Brooklyn Mall in Pretoria. “Practitioners” span a broad spectrum of practices. And, although covering a range of diverse practices, it is useful to identify two main categories of traditional practitioners. First, there are *diviner-diagnosticians* (also called diviner-mediums), who give diagnosis through spiritual means. Second, there are *healers*, or *herbalists*, who choose and supply remedies on the basis of a diagnosis (Berger and Heywood 2007).[1] These are the two main categories confirmed from fieldwork but that in practice are often hard to distinguish. In particular, the use of herbs or similar remedies, based on consultation with healers, often involving rolling bones and “reading” them, is the form of traditional medication most commonly referred to in this chapter. This is not to be confused with the broad range of products and alternative medications that also feature very prominently in accounts by people living with AIDS in this area, although sometimes the lines can appear quite blurred.

“Alternative” treatments are advertised particularly vigorously, amounting to a rapidly growing economic sector. A bewildering range of products has come to the fore. These appear to colonize spaces of uncertainty surrounding the disputed science of AIDS in South Africa. The scale of the problem can be gauged by looking at Figure 6.1. It typically depicts products for sale at a supermarket, whether Hammanskraal, inner-city areas, or in Hoedespruit, where the image was actually taken.

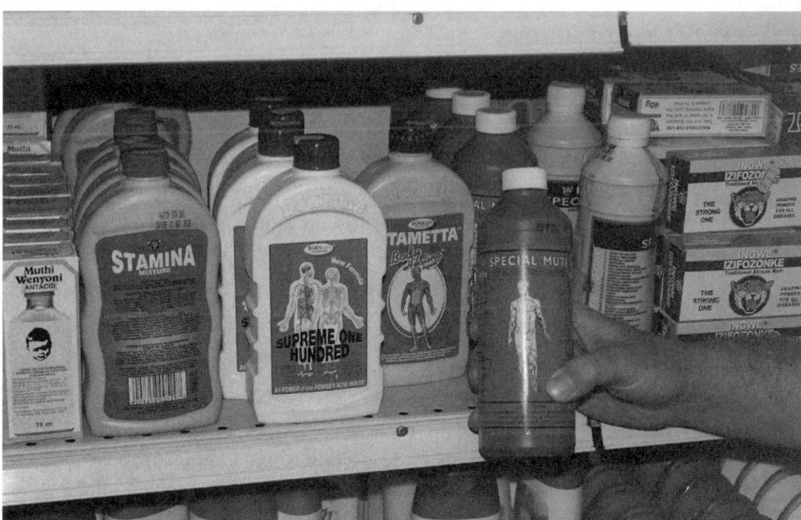

Figure 6.1 “Alternative” treatments in store

The photo shows how such areas have become competitive arenas for alternative products. A range of products can be seen. Many of these brand names—for example, *Muti*—although "alternative" products nonetheless, evoke more traditionalist sentiments of the consumer.[2] Products vary from those based on herbal remedies to those representing "immune boosters" or some combination of both. Some of them explicitly claim on the packaging to treat AIDS. The chapter seeks out some of the reasons for the allure of traditional and alternative treatment and, above all, implications of such a challenge to ARVs. Additionally, public health and rights-based approaches to AIDS and AIDS treatment, despite self-professed protestations to the contrary, often end up regarding culture, at worst, as a barrier to modern medicine that needs eradication, or, at best, that should be regulated in accordance with their own preferred image. Or, alternatively, perhaps culture is simply totally ignored, a nonstarter for discussion.

One comprehensive academic overview of AIDS in South Africa, for example, even describing itself as "definitive," draws on scientific, biological, political, and social science dimensions of the epidemic. But for all this there is a glaring omission: in this tome spanning some 600 pages there appears to be extremely limited space given to discussion of cultural constructions of AIDS. Despite drawing our attention to the important role of alternative disease constructs, this topic receives mention on only a couple of pages in total (Abdool Karim and Abdul Karim (2005:486, 487, 536). There is little beyond flagging its existence and then a call for "some form of cooperation with, if not cooption of complementary traditional health care system."[3] It appears to be an opportunity lost for engagement with cultural aspects of AIDS. This deficit is all the more pronounced as public health interventions are negotiating exactly these same aspects that may be conditioning their outcomes. Alternatively, some researcher-activists do invoke these cultural dimensions or at least affirm them as having a potentially positive role. Importantly, some of the better and more sensitive work highlights exploitation of vulnerable people and how "culture" is not static but can be open to abusive and harmful unregulated practices (Berger and Heywood 2007). Other research locates the challenges of controlling the epidemic within a need to create awareness of the role of cultural perceptions. Not least, this is because such perceptions may lead to explanations and treatments that may be ineffective or that even exacerbate transmission of the virus (Golooba-Mutebi and Tollman 2007). Both dimensions are explored in this chapter. But, nonetheless, there is still a tendency to regard culture as in need of aligning itself with either public health or a rights-based approach, which resonates more broadly with dilemmas in reconciling culture and rights (see Chapter 2). Certainly, in the context of bogus science, denialism, and peddling of quack remedies, culture is being used in order to abuse vulnerable people living with HIV/AIDS. But, beyond this misuse within communities like Hammanskraal, what is then nonetheless the continuing resilient appeal of traditional and alternative medication?

Confused Communities

How an elite-driven focus has imprinted itself upon traditional and alternative medication in the context of a search for African-made "alternatives" to ARVs and, indeed, explanations of the epidemic itself, was shown in previous chapters. In mapping out the interplay between top-down agendas and bottom-up realities, one issue is whether government has actually followed its agenda and supported clarity, definition over practices, and especially, policy and funding for initiatives to implement it. Otherwise, is the role envisaged by key politicians for the inclusion of "African alternatives" in the context of HIV/AIDS at odds with the reality? That this inclusion has gained momentum is beyond doubt. This is evident in the creation of an expert Committee on African Traditional Medicine. Furthermore, key scientific research and regulatory bodies, such as the Council for Scientific and Industrial Research, the Medical Research Council, and the Department of Health are involved in collating a database of plant-related medications. As previously mentioned, the role of traditional medication was envisaged in its own chapter in the operational plan (see Chapter 1). Another development was the creation of a pharmacovigilance center[4] to monitor properties of traditional products, amongst other things, and adverse effects for ARVs. While these can be considered positive steps in developing efforts to monitor the potential, efficacy, and safety of traditional and alternative medications, there appears to be a vacuum in funding. And, it is especially concerning whether reliable information exists at a grassroots level in order to inform patients of choices in medication.

Monna wa maledu, for example, refers locally to an African potato in Hammanskraal/Temba. Members of an AIDS hospice support group, who, whilst claiming it was similar to the African potato, nonetheless identified it as also having different properties.[5] Heated debate and opinions were traded in this group. Indeed, confusion reigned about the different types of African potato in two of the focus groups, notably underscored by appeals for clarity:

> We have misunderstanding in our community. You see, for example, I can say the minister of health, she used to say "you must use the African potato," you see, and then we as black people we know that African potato is that black thing with some roots. We use them but it's not the one they were talking about. You see there are different types of African potatoes. The other thing is that it makes your stomach run. The other African potato we usually have to find. Even when

> our African doctors go out and look for traditional herbs they will come up with that African potato. They must use the other one because even the color is not the same. That one is dark green . . . the other one is light. We misunderstand them. Then we use the wrong thing, you see. ("Thando")

This confusion would appear even more significant given that the Department of Health's own information cautions against use of African potato because it decreases the efficacy of ARVs (see next section). These comments also make a direct—unprompted—connection with the minister of health, and the Africanist agenda of key sections of the government, as mentioned. The role of leaders in shaping certain perceptions of ARVs was suggested in the previous chapter. And it is important to note that what the minister or others who are part of this agenda say does filter down to local communities like Temba. In terms of other "alternative" products, such as the lemon, garlic, olive oil, and African potato mixture prompted by the minister of health, another group also expressed confusion:

> *"Rose":* In the Wellness workshop they tell us to take garlic but only until one starts taking ARVs. Once you take the ARVs you should stop taking garlic but then the health Minister says you should continue taking garlic.
> *Facilitator:* But, what do you think?
> *"Wandi":* we don't know. We are confused.

While the depth and spread of traditional and alternative medication cannot solely be attributed to the elitist Africanist nation-building project, it undoubtedly contributes to sowing the seeds of confusion in this community. The contested nature of ARVs and the generally negative debates about them and broader explanations of HIV/AIDS itself surely play into already-existing strong local belief systems. But it would be a mistake to regard use of either as mutually exclusive. What appears more accurate is how traditional and alternative medication *co-exists* with the ARV era and within what others have described as a double or even triple layering of consciousness (Robins 2005). Evidence of "layering" was reflected especially in respondents' common assertions of their mixing of different medication.

To Mix or Not to Mix Medication

It became apparent that at least several participants openly revealed use of herbs (and other products), typically used alongside ARVs: "Yes, I also take ARVs with herbs. It does not do me any harm. I don't even suffer from stress" ("Nonni"). And a male in the same group said: "When I started using ARVs, I was told to use only ARVs and not to mix them with any other thing for the first four months. The first four months, I took only ARVs . . . they [unclear who] encouraged me to take herbs. Now I am using herbs but then I am still taking ARVs. They told me how to use the herbs" ("Thando"). And another male said about alternative products: "I have seen many people being helped by these—they call it "natural health'" [nature's health]. They helped many people . . . so I'm convinced that they are doing the work [i.e., beneficial]" ("Sibo"). Another participant, "Thando," in the same group nonetheless claimed, "but we as a people, I don't know, I feel sometimes because . . . people I meet they will say 'no, traditional herbs work more than ARVs.'" But the issue of coexistence of different medicines revealed itself repeatedly in the context of debates over the desirability of mixing ARVs and traditional products. For example, "Nonni" exemplified this practice: "I think that most of the times many of us take ARVs and mix them with other treatment. Some of us have not even started taking ARVs and when we start taking ARVs and mix some, people start saying that these things are not working." Although it was denied by the clinic, some respondents felt that information given was ambiguous:

> We do not know the truth. For instance, if I can go to a doctor now and say I have TB and I am HIV positive, can I use any boosters and he says no but when I go to the other doctor he will say yes. We are not getting the truth and we do not know what to do. What I think is that one should use what is working for him and not mix them rather than copying what other people are using. I don't see the reason why they should use herbs because ARVs are boosters. People should stick to what works for them. ("Thando")

Again, the level of confusion was apparent with another woman making an appeal for clarification: "How about we find someone to come and clarify to us? I was told that you are not supposed to mix, some mix" ("Rose"). Others also suggested the practice was even more widespread because "people hide themselves, you can't see that they take both ARVs and traditional medication." Another claimed that "really there are more people taking both ARVs and traditional medication because when it's the time to do [ARVs] medication they just go . . . [to the bathroom]."

There was also a generational aspect to this secrecy. Some parents do not want their children to take ARVs. Instead, according to the leader of a home-based care organization, despite protestations from children, the latter acquiesce to using herbs although they may still take ARVs secretly. "T," a key informant member of the clinic support group suggested that many others in the group did not wish to come forward as taking traditional medication. However, even within that particular group, many were mixing medication, he claimed. This group was based at a hospice in Temba. Herbs were available for purchase at this hospice and occasionally other products were offered for sale to people living with AIDS. Before asking if there are any benefits, the question of whether there are any particular problems with this use of traditional medication is first posed.

"It's Business Now"

An entry point into answering this question of whether there are particular problems associated with traditional medication is to cite one member of the Sunrise hospice support group. This person claimed that most members at the hospice would buy whatever product was available in the desperate hope they will be cured. Even *Mopane* worms were at one point claimed to have healing properties and bought by hospice members. This illustrates the broader national context whereby communities are flooded with treatments and miracle cures, marketed quite vigorously and targeting vulnerable people. Even the head of Wellness, Dr. Mathibedi, had himself been approached by a company called "Nature's Health" to promote their herbal product to his patients. If he endorsed their product, he was told, Dr. Mathibedi, "could be made a rich man" by Nature's Health. These developments indicate that alternative treatments in South Africa have become a big industry—some estimates put the value at over two billion rand per year (Berger and Heywood 2007). That this community is awash with unregulated and unproven medications merely compounds the situation. The community is bombarded with all kinds of medication. There is the danger, however, in dealing with any vulnerable group that they will be exposed to unethical and immoral exploitation.

The significant challenge posed to ARVs by traditional medication was verified by the clinic. Dr. Mathibedi, for example, observed how, when they first come to the clinic, the majority of patients bring something called *Immunodu*, a combination of herbs and multivitamins. All people living with AIDS focus groups mentioned these products. In general, they appeared to be widely used. Use of products like this is discouraged by the clinic because, it was explained, rather than spending R100 on products such as *Immunodu*, patients can get free multivitamins and ARVs from the clinic themselves. Second, the herbs in this product, like others, contain traces of African potato, which, according to Wellness itself can present problems for ARV resistance. Another respondent mentioned a friend who died after taking herbs. Despite showing some awareness of the dangers about mixing medications, this persisted: "If you take herbs and ARVs and there is a problem in your body, they will not be able to identify the problem in your body. But if you take ARVs, they can maybe say AZT is not good for you and find another drug for you because there are many drugs. I don't know how [the hospital] is operating but the law is supposed to stop one from mixing these things" ("Rose").

However, "T," for example, mentioned at least ten acquaintances that, in recent years, had mixed both ARVs and herbs, which led him to comment that: "I can tell you and assure [you] that all those people are no longer existing. They are dead, they passed away." From January 2006 to the time of the interview in July of that year, six people at this local community AIDS hospice alone had passed away. Most, it was claimed, arose apparently due to mixing medication and/or interrupting ARV use for other reasons, sometimes financial (see next chapter). So, some participants knew the risks of mixing medication. But that there was so much discussion and conflicting opinions (particularly in the hospice-based group) indicates a large degree of confusion and the persistence with traditional medications despite knowing the dangers.

The clinic appears to take a very pragmatic view. People living with AIDS are given a choice, based on information about each type of product. This, I was told, is in order not to alienate those patients using traditional or alternative medication. The choice also includes information to make patients aware of the potential conflict between ARVs and alternatives that can impede the efficacy and that may be harmful. This approach appears in line with the national information on treatment provided by the Department of Health's *Khomamani* campaign, as discussed in Chapter 1. This campaign indicates a clash between different treatments and emphasizes that herbs and traditional medication can affect the efficacy of ARVs. In the respondent groups, opinions, however, were varied and more open-ended. Whereas some would say patients should not mix them, another would respond typically: "me, the way I know it, you can take ARVs with a herbal treatment because they have no side effects." Others suggested that the real problem was not the herbs *per se* but rather the inaccurate dosages with traditional herbs because there were vague limits on how much one should use. Another aspect was that peoples' desire to heal quickly led them to disregard advice on the appropriate dosage.[6]

The role of traditional healers was therefore cited as particularly significant. Widespread confusion is evident about the different types of traditional medication and, in related fashion, defining appropriate doses for patients. Several types of medication were mentioned in focus group discussions. There were often conflicting views on various types of treatment. This confirms nationwide patterns of health-seeking behavior in that a person is more likely to first approach a *Sangoma* before the hospital as last resort. Indeed, the number of black South Africans approaching traditional healers is estimated by the Department of Health itself as at least 70 percent. Sadly, however, as alluded to, the room for nuanced debate on the role of traditional medication and healers has tended to be squeezed out. It had fallen hostage, instead, first to colonial and apartheid era modernist views viewing African tradition as inferior. Second, more recently, post-apartheid nation-building has sought to reify values considered to offer something more Afro-centered to counter the previous discourse that denigrated African culture and tradition. "Tradition" and culture continue to be a political football. Hence, the claims for its beneficial use, as with those for ARVs, have become polarized, stuck in binary opposition.

The previous head of Wellness, for example, referred to one patient who, upon the advice of a traditional healer, stopped using ARVs because he had wanted to "feel strong" when appearing in a court case. When the case was resolved (he lost it), he restarted ARVs. Dr. Mathibedi also referred to the influence of healers upon another patient. After checking the blood results of the patient who had stopped improving from use of ARVs, it was subsequently discovered that the patient's traditional healer had told him to stop taking ARVs. Both heads of Wellness highlighted the problem of interrupted use of ARVs when patients use traditional medication and how this can contribute to resistance and lower absorption of ARVs with which to hold the virus in check. So, in addition to mixing, interrupting treatment at particular junctures in a patients' life is another practice.

"Wandi" also raised the role of traditional healers in convincing patients to interrupt ARV treatment: "They [her cousins' parents] said that they have a problem with the ancestors, since he is in the initiation to become a *Sangoma*. They think that it has to do with that since he is in initiation he stopped going to the clinic and taking the medication." Several respondents claimed that too many people in their community were dying because of these practices. How, then, do we seek to explain the use of traditional medication?

Explaining Traditional Medication

Thando's comments, in the quotation below, provide some clues in seeking to explain the allure of alternative conceptions of illness and traditional medication. Thando refers to allure locally as *Makhome*: "There is that mindset of, eh! old things, that most of the people still do not believe that HIV. It is what we call in our language *Makhome*. I don't know what it is called in English but that thing can be cured but traditional healers can only cure it. They have that belief." *Makhome* can therefore be identified as one of four distinct categories of perceived explanations of illness identified by researchers. The first concerns natural causes and God-given explanations. The second refers to eating certain foods too often or in large quantities. Witchcraft comprises another category, with human agency involved whereby someone is fed (in a dream or real life) with something poisonous that is "injurious to their health." Finally, there is an explanation for ill health, related to two types of pollution. One is the belief, according to Golooba-Mutebi and Tollman (2007:117), in environmental pollution such as dust that is believed to cause TB in miners and ex-miners. The other is ritual-based and relates to particular customs or traditions that have been violated. In this case, *Makhome* is not in fact witchcraft[7] but rather illness explained by the transgression of taboos. *Makhome* is related in particular to the violation of the custom of a spouse abstaining from sex in a defined period following the death of a husband or wife. Some of the symptoms of *Makhome* described in Hammanskraal include swelling legs, coughing, and bleeding (Zuberi et al 2004).

Witchcraft, regarded as a significant explanation of HIV/AIDS, has been mentioned in the context of previous fieldwork. In that report (Zuberi et al 2004), in the context of exploring reasons for stigma, the negative connotations associated with witchcraft were certainly identified as contributing to stigmatization. "Thando," for example, described the power of belief in witchcraft in explanation if AIDS-related illness:

> This issue of HIV is also associated with witchcraft. If a person is facing terminally ill stage, they will relate it to witchcraft. They will argue that "the signs are similar to witchcraft." That is why most of the time they take a sick person to a traditional healer because they think he was bewitched, they don't want to consider the fact that it is HIV/AIDS. They just say it is witchcraft because they see symptoms of a person who was bewitched. As a result, they don't want to be closer to that person because they think those things that are in him will be transmitted to them. Like witchcraft, as we know witchcraft is a spirit, no matter how you teach them about this thing, they will not trust you because of witchcraft. So this is what gives them a problem about HIV.

Witchcraft therefore shifts the explanation of causes of HIV/AIDS from the realm of biology and evidence-based medicine to more supernatural factors. When someone died of AIDS, it was often attributed to someone having cast a spell on them. Symptoms such as burning feet and legs were deemed to mean someone having buried something in the ground, putting a curse on the person. Golooba and Tollman refer to this as *Xidyiso* whereas a Tswana term used locally in Hammanskraal-Temba refers to it as *Sejiso*. Many respondents referred to such practices. Witchcraft is of course a product of the social world in which people live, comprising and comprised by specific social, economic, and political events. And that social world in Hammanskraal/Temba is a harsh one, characterized, as it is, by high unemployment, poverty, hardship, fear of AIDS-related morality and illness, and development that appears sloth-like. Seen in this light, if we are to even attempt to get close to comprehending its significant role in the context of contemporary South Africa, it is more appropriate and constructive to view witchcraft as related to broader anxieties, fears, and paradoxes of the post-apartheid era. To reiterate some of these from Chapter 1, on the one hand, freedoms and opportunities have multiplied, but so has deeper insecurity and perceptions that those freedoms and rights, on the other, have displaced tradition and authority (Posel et al 2007). People seek to rationalize their shifting fortunes, particularly the onset of misfortune. These are the local worldviews that need to be understood and decoded in more detail than can be granted here. But a fundamental issue that is directly relevant is how health-seeking behavior—including use of ARVs—must simultaneously negotiate both tradition and modernity. So, are such beliefs merely harmless coping mechanisms to negotiate post-apartheid insecurities, particularly in explaining the huge increase in AIDS-related mortality? Or, do some beliefs associated with harmful practices directly contribute to mortality and expose vulnerable groups to harm?

First, "Minkie," for example, viewed *Sejiso* in the context of parental decision-making over children she and other home-based carers encountered daily through their work. She alluded to a distinct generational aspect to beliefs and whether ARVs are deemed appropriate:

> But you can see that this child, this poor child [is] supposed to go to the hospital. And some of them just cough. They just cough, cough, cough, and throw the spit out, cough and throw the spit out. And the spit, when I look at it, has little clots of blood. You can see that this is TB. But they [the traditional healer] say that they can cure it. "*Sejiso*," they say, something like, if you treat and eat ["Western" medication] it damages inside your chest. That is not true . . . I'm telling you that is not good. I was saying that maybe another thing that the government must do is something about the traditional healer or give us the right to go and take that little poor child. I do not know what I'm supposed to do about that because it is not good at all, it is not good. ("Minkie")[8]

Intense frustration was expressed concerning diagnostic practices like *Sejiso* whereby children were placed in vulnerable, health-damaging positions by parents who subscribe to such beliefs. In another case, a traditional healer gave ARVs, as well as herbs, to one patient respondent. But she was given both only after the healer requested the patient produce a test notification from clinic. The quality of linkages between traditional healers and mainstream health services would therefore appear critical. In some cases, for instance, local healers who were interviewed claimed not to diagnose or treat a person for AIDS before they produced a test certificate. In the case of these local Sangomas, in fact, a mother and son whose clients came from as far away as Johannesburg, HIV/AIDS was regarded as a combination of illnesses that can be cured. They claimed they could tell whether a person is HIV-positive by touching the veins and looking at their tongue. They would throw the bones to determine if blood is black, and if it was black, HIV was suspected. Despite evidence of some sort of arrangement with referring people to the hospital for testing, they nonetheless claimed to have cured four people.[9] This suggests that some healers maintain fundamental differences in interpreting and treating AIDS-related illness.

Second, just as there are many good and reputable Sangomas, there are many who are not and who may be tempted by profiteering and to be more exploitative of their patients. With some Sangomas apparently claiming they could cure AIDS for up to R1500, the link with business and economic exploitation of people living with AIDS has become all too apparent. Other abuses concerned, when, in peoples' desperation to be cured, a Sangoma allegedly wanted sex with his patients as part of the curative process. In relation to this, and a previous quote concerning someone's relative who was training to be a Sangoma, "Minkie" also cited the increasing popularity of training to become a *Sangoma*. This was, she claimed, to do with a mistaken belief that one could be healed in the process. But practices involved in the training were considered harmful. Some cited included cutting the skin with a razor blade in order to release "bad" blood through a "cleansing" process. Another involved the inhalation of smoke, which may exacerbate chest-related conditions.

Third, a fundamental issue raised by respondents is therefore the critical time period lost to initiating ARVs because of the time taken to consult and be treated by a Sangoma:

> Because you know what I have realized . . . is that one day that traditional healer realizes that now there is nothing they can do about this patient. That patient spends lots of time there, they tried all their traditional medication, and then there is nothing they can do. When you come with your parents they say "eish, just take the patient. There is nothing I can do." And you start fighting with lots of words. Difficult words [i.e., angry and confused]. After that, you take the child. And you want to take that child now to the hospital, you see. That is why at hospital they say "there is nothing we can do so take this medication and go." And when you go home you find us [i.e., approach the home-based carers] now. You want us to take care of the children while we have told you from the beginning don't take this child to the traditional healer. Just allow the hospital to take care of the child by providing her with ARVs but you said "no we will take her there," you see. ("Minkie")

Given that there is a significant problem in South Africa with many people living with AIDS approaching ARV services only at a late stage of illness, this is a critical area for review and intervention.

Other types of medication mentioned included *Ubhejani*, the "medication" that had been unofficially promoted by the minister of health at the time and an influential network behind its production in KwaZulu Natal. Respondents had raised questions about this treatment with the clinic in the belief that it worked. The connection between government and these products was firmly identified as follows: "Since they discovered HIV/AIDS, there are so many mortuaries that have been opened and even boosters [alternative products]. It is business now. Even the government has approved a lot of things. People are now confused. *They say that because these things have been approved by the government we have to take them*" ("Gloria"; emphasis added). Again, this illustrates how the official discourse surrounding alternatives to ARVs does influence patient choices and mingles with already existing views on explaining and treating AIDS.

Another treatment was cited that is more closely related to spiritual beliefs and the spiritual prophets of the Church of Zion (ZCC). This included the ZCC's "*strong coffee*": "He [the brother who was mentioned in the previous chapter regarding denial and AIDS] takes some strong coffee at a ZCC church. Now I've seen that he has lost a lot of weight. When I speak to him he says he is going to stop taking that traditional medication but he hasn't yet stopped." Members of ZCC also cited the importance of bathing rituals as part of the spiritual cleansing of HIV. One in particular was highly critical of traditional practices while seeing no conflict with ZCC practices. There was clearly an undertone of some practicing Christians of the undesirability of traditional approaches. In this case, however, it was also suggested that such ZCC practices should not be to the exclusion of ARVs. But again, coexistence of treatment appears most likely.

While some dubious practices and effects associated with traditional treatment have been mentioned, there are undoubtedly some benefits, not least because they refer to patient's cosmological outlook and, hence, cultural acceptability.

Benefits of Traditional Medication

Traditional medication was identified as having several benefits. First, focus groups mentioned, for example, that contrary to delaying hospital or clinic care, seeking traditional medication was actually an important first stage in accepting ones own HIV status. This was described as: "I have to start somewhere and if I have to start somewhere already I'm engaging myself to traditional herbs" ("Thando"). In other words, traditional medicine could be an important entry point to seeking, or being referred to, the ARV clinic but at an early stage.

Second, another factor given was that there was less anxiety associated with herbs than with the strict time management of ARVs:

> I think at first, like I said, I didn't want to take the ARVs. The thing was I have seen these herbs helping people. Then I was asking myself, after they told me that the ARVs are for life, you understand, then if it is for life, then the time management, again it's a problem. Then I compared the two, because they told me to take one of them. It's either the herbs or the ARVs. So the person who is taking herbs won't run the risk of time management, because if you take, let's say, a cup in the morning, then it's fine. But with the ARVs you must be punctual, 8 o'clock in the morning 8 o'clock in the evening. ("Sibo")

In a related fashion, given the identification in an earlier chapter of fears over side effects, patients may rationalize that they have been told that alternatives have the same function as ARVs. But because they believe that traditional medication does not have side effects, this is a sort of "win-win" situation, hedging bets, if you like. The result is that they can take both—with associated risks previously mentioned—or interrupt ARV use. It also places the clinic in an awkward position because they must balance between stressing the possibility of side effects to prepare the patient for this and to enable a more positive response, yet they do not wish to discourage patients from using ARVs.

It was also identified as a product of the family culture whereby this was regarded as a more acceptable channel for seeking help. It was described as legitimated because this "timeless" type of medication has helped grandparents and parents for decades. Furthermore, there is also the aspect that while ARVs are free, the family may have already paid for traditional medication and this should be finished first. So, traditional medication was deemed by many to be more culturally acceptable. However, as stated, there was additional evidence of generational pressure, with the older generation pressuring children into taking traditional medication.

Others also pointed out that given the stigmatization associated by ARVs with AIDS, traditional alternatives removed the stigma because observers did not know what the person was being treated for, at least, or reduced the signification of AIDS: "Because most of people they mix it. The other ones prefer to drink the traditional medication because if he drinks it no one can realize that you are HIV positive. Everyone can drink it" ("T"). Interestingly, it may also be less stigmatized to have a "traditional illness" rather than AIDS, although fear was evident concerning witchcraft-related illness. In the meeting with the Sangoma, it was noticeable how they never referred to "HIV/AIDS," and chose to place it within the realm of "traditional illness," a result of displeasing ancestors or transgressing taboos. The apparent lack of judgment of patients and stigmatization was in stark contrast, it must be said, to discriminatory patient treatment at Jubilee hospital (Chapter 4). While this of course begs the question of whether ARVs can be perceived as positive in such a traditional paradigm, it does appear to remove the stigma associated with labels such as HIV/AIDS. While it may be harmful to ARV use, why, in the first place, patients perceive traditional healers as more acceptable must be recognized.

In terms of the questionnaire, it was noticeable that no respondent mentioned they were using traditional or alternative medication. But, interestingly, only six of twenty respondents gave any response at all: five stated "no," and the sixth remarked, "traditional medication can't heal." It begs the question of why this was the most unanswered section of the questionnaire. This is undoubtedly a reflection of the constrained environment within which the questionnaire was given by the ARV clinic social worker. Perhaps this influenced the participants to give the "right" answer or, in terms of traditional medication, no answer. But it does nonetheless show that this group has had considerable exposure to information about ARVs. This seems to be in marked contrast to the community as a whole. Furthermore, even if not mentioned in the questionnaire, use of herbs was clearly stated by many within focus groups.

With such competition from traditional and alternative treatments and indeed given the general level of confusion about the desirability or otherwise of mixing different treatments, and in explanations of illness, inevitably some people are being filtered out from access to ARV treatment. The chapter has shown that "tradition" and "culture" are not intrinsically benevolent. There is not necessarily even any definitive agreement on what the cultural practices are. Culture is not neutral. Other research shows, for example, how traditional healers have a very influential role in upholding cultural norms also surrounding procreation (in explaining and treating infertility) that serve to reinforce the subordinate social roles of women. Traditional healer explanations of infertility and illness and adverse well being of children are especially attributed to women breaking traditional codes of conduct and committing adultery, unlike men, whose adultery and polygamy is tolerated (Hellum 1999).

And some practices can be both abused by practitioners and abusive and outright unacceptable to patients. This does raise the specter of the urgent need for regulation in the context of AIDS "treatments." At the same time, however, regarding culture as merely something from which to extract properties and information to make products from herbs, or to regulate it, tends to belittle the deep symbolism, belonging, and power of local world views. This may be an inevitable trade off. But it is one that should be minimized so that we do not lose sight of the cultural attachments people have. One implication is that health services and ARV clinics should strive to be culturally acceptable wherever possible. A public health and rights-based approach must seek to identify when something is considered culturally acceptable or unacceptable. Regulation is clearly needed but it should not be to the detriment of genuine cultural practices and, above all, recognition of the existence of plural systems for health-seeking behavior. The clinic at Wellness is attempting to negotiate these cultural issues and appears to have adopted a highly pragmatic approach. But there is still plenty of scope for better interaction between so-called evidence-based and traditional health systems. Not least, the cultural confidence of communities, like Hammanskraal/Temba must be still be won. And part of this undoubtedly lies in providing coherent, consistent information that must be given on both ARVs and traditional medicine so that communities can make informed choices about treatment. But it is also very much about fashioning a better co-existence between these different health care systems.

The next chapter looks at additional barriers in access—those that are more structural and that are associated with the process to initiate treatment itself at the local clinic.

CHAPTER 7

Accessing Treatment

Socioeconomic Issues and Clinic Criteria

Jubilee, they want many things before you can get ARVs.

—"Thandi"

The human right to health, including treatment, as shown in Chapter 2, usefully serves to identify barriers that obstruct access to services and the principled measures needed to overcome them. Previous chapters have been concerned with placing these barriers within the broader political, cultural, and social landscape within Hammanskraal/Temba. In addition, the significant role played by socioeconomic factors is now gaining the recognition deserved in studies of treatment programs. Since research for the book began in Hammanskraal/Temba, across all people interviewed, focus groups and informal discussions held, when asked about key characteristics of the area, most—if not almost all—associate it with high levels of poverty and unemployment. Unemployment is endemic, particularly among school-leavers and younger people. Another key and related dynamic concerns dismissals from work, poor job security, and problems with receiving employment-related payouts such as pensions. Often, links were also made between poverty, joblessness, and vulnerability to HIV/AIDS.

In such a context, it should appear necessary to explore what challenges are posed by the political economy of the area to ARV programs and in realizing human rights more generally. This chapter therefore seeks to contribute to this broader discussion of the specific barriers posed to ARV programs by socioeconomic circumstances. This chapter explores whether the ARV program in Hammanskraal/Temba sufficiently takes into account this context, which, for some patients, as in the quotation above, manifests itself as Jubilee "want[ing] many things before you can get ARVs."

And in relation to specific requirements, the treatment selection and preparation process "wants" of patients, in light of previous discussion of the importance of criteria in access, where such criteria emerged as topics in focus groups, these are mentioned. The role of disclosure and ethical issues in selection criteria to access treatment is especially important to gauge. Above all, who is getting and not getting access to medication and what difficulties are being encountered are considered.

Who Is Finding It Difficult to Access ARVs?

In addition to the broad figures presented in Table 4.1 in Chapter 4, the question of which groups were finding it hardest to access medication was put to the clinic patient support group. It is felt that although this group is a captured sample in the sense of being from the same support group and perhaps reflecting attitudes related to membership of the group, this was a good representative sample, drawn, as it was, from across a broad geographical catchment area of Wellness. There was an ambiguous response in identifying specific groups but "rural dwellers," "poor," "unemployed," and those described as "in denial" were all especially highlighted in responses. And those encountering "denial," of course, may not necessarily be confined to those other categories. In terms of getting better statistical verification of the questionnaire, the following responses were collated. Of those responses given by the eighteen respondents answering, the most commonly identified category is shown first in Table 7.1.

Significantly, it appears that specific individual vulnerable groups—man having sex with men, prisoners, etc.—tend not to be identified as those encountering particular difficulties in accessing ARVs. Only one specific group is named, "school children," although, as stated, respondents mention the "poor," "unemployed," and "rural" as perhaps encountering more difficulties. Perhaps it is possible to qualify these responses with the respondent's tendency to identify

Table 7.1 Who finds it hard to access ARVs according to clinic support group?

Category most commonly stated by respondents	*Percentage responses*
"No one/not hard"	25%
"People in rural area/destitute/poor/unemployed"	20%
"Those not knowing status and/or in denial"	20%
"Many"	5%
"Those not following rules of hospital"	5%
"Those fearful of ARVs"	5%
"School children"	5%
Other	15%

more personal factors such as one's attitude and the role of personal responsibility. This may explain why a particularly large number of responses cited either "no one" or still "in denial" and "not knowing their status." Perhaps this reflects their perception that access is possible but contingent upon taking responsibility and acceptance, like they themselves had done. Similarly, "no one" in particular may relate to no one special, implying, again, it is the role of personal convictions and determination in accessing treatment that means that others can or should do it. The responses most likely reflect the phenomenon of actually being in a support group and feeling like they have undergone some kind of conversion in accepting their status, or at least coming to terms with it, often associated in particular with near-death experiences, which separates them from the "other" (i.e., those not accepting or knowing status). Either way, it still shows the scale of the obstacle posed by personal denial.

Is it Easy or Hard to Access?

The questionnaire also asked about the process involved in accessing treatment. To make this more statistically verifiable, the questionnaire (also translated into Setswana) posed the following to the treatment support group: "To get access to ARVs, is it: a) easy b) not difficult c) hard d) very hard e) nearly impossible." Of nineteen responses, the following were recorded:

A) 37 percent
B) 26 percent
C) 16 percent
D) 0 percent
E) 21 percent

Therefore, the clear majority, 63 percent, felt it was easy or at least not too difficult to access treatment. However, 37 percent did think it was difficult or impossible to get access. Can we correlate these responses with other factors?

Well, of this latter category, of those most likely to reply "c" or "e," over 70 percent are also likely to live outside of the "core" residential area around the hospital. The role of geography here is obvious. For example, of those Wellness support group respondents, residence is as follows: 40 percent live in Wards 74 or 75 (not always made clear but assumed to be relatively close in Temba); 25 percent in Ward 73 (Hammanskraal and some surrounding villages); 15 percent in the Makapanstad area (i.e., over 20km away, in the North West province); and 10 percent in Ward 8 (also particularly far, including 10 percent in the Soshanguve/Stinkwater area). Distance from point of access is therefore an important codeterminant in accessing treatment.

Other Socioeconomic Factors

Again, in terms of the questionnaire, responses seemed to cross over categories the questionnaire had hoped to group them under. For example, responses to questions on "access," "adherence," as well as "additional suggestions," seemed not to discern discreet categories but rather crossed all of them. So, whereas if we take the question aimed at identifying the most common factors making it difficult to adhere, for example, time management appears to be the most frequent response. This was then followed by economic issues, equal to both side effects and "attitude/denial/knowledge," with two then stating social problems and lack of family support. But because, as mentioned, there is such crossover of responses beyond these discreet categories of "access," "adherence," and "additional suggestions," it was decided to combine these into one group. Therefore, responses could be grouped around the following themes, with the main one being that: *70 percent of respondents identified a range of socioeconomic and related service delivery issues across all the categories—access, adherence, and in citing additional factors.*

The context of political economy appears to weigh heavily. These concerns were stated as follows, in order of the most commonly cited. First, food, money, and transport were all cited most and equally significantly. Second, these were followed by the importance of bringing treatment closer to the people living with AIDS through decentralization of ARV access points to local communities. Third, also cited, again in decreasing significance, social grants, clean water (particularly important for one rural dweller), and costs involved in eating healthy. Fourth, transport is another major issue, as mentioned, with 66 percent of those specifically citing it, also living outside of the "core" area of the hospital. One respondent from Makapanstad, for example, mentioned the burden of having to travel 23km to Wellness clinic when they did not have money to do this regularly. But this was still an important issue even for the approximately 37 percent citing it as significant, yet, who lived relatively closer. Finally, many mentioned the importance of food as a major challenge in taking ARVs, specifically in the context of the harm and nausea in taking them on an empty stomach.

It is therefore important to interpret the socioeconomic criteria and recommendations of decentralized ARV service points as an interrelated set of structural issues difficult to disentangle. Many respondents, for example, cite "money" and/or "food" and "transport" separately, whereas these are interrelated and often due to lack of income. Therefore, although three residents specifically mention social grants, perhaps more may have this in mind when citing "money," "food," and "transport" difficulties. Similarly, respondents citing decentralization of ARV sites to a more localized point of access most likely do so due to the burden and costs of transport and vice versa. Therefore, it is considered here that it is important to focus on the aggregate impact of these factors, as reflected in them being cited by 70 percent of respondents. This figure also tends to reinforce the census data information shown in Chapter 3, which depicted the high level of socioeconomic deprivation across this area.

Had the question perhaps been expressed more clearly and administered differently, if anything, then the level of respondents identifying socio-conomic issues might have been even higher (i.e., they might have felt less inclined to recite treatment preparation information had the social worker not been there). For all the shortcomings of the questionnaire, it does tend, nonetheless, to reinforce the critical role of socioeconomic circumstances in accessing, and then once accessed, ability to adhere to ARVs. The following discussions from the focus groups and interviews add more qualitative insights.

The focus groups also raised the role of socioeconomic circumstances prominently. It quickly became apparent that transport was critical as a key issue for many. One woman, for example, cited transport as follows: "Okay then, yah! My problem concerns money for transport [from home to the clinic]. We do not have the money. For instance, I have to go today and then after two days I have to go again. We do not have the money. You skip your treatment and when you have money you go there and they tell you that your date has already passed." That this may lead to "skipping treatment" is of great concern for adherence. Of ten patients who the clerk tells the social worker do not come on a given day, typically, she says that nine of these are due to lack of transport money. The obvious issue of distance was important, and this chimes with the questionnaire findings that problems arise when one cannot walk to the clinic:

> *"Thandi":* You cannot walk from your place of residence to the hospital.
> *Facilitator:* So you miss appointments, for example?
> *"Thandi":* Yah! I do miss appointments. Last month, for example, I was supposed to go on the 12th but I was having a financial problem. Then I go to the clinic and explain to them. Then they give me a letter and then I go to the Wellness clinic and explain to them that I have missed my treatment because I had a financial problem."

"T" had to travel even further to receive his treatment. He spoke about his own transport problems:

> It affects me a lot. But there are people who usually sometimes help me, they borrow me money. Like now, there is still some people I owe them, I'm not able to pay them back, because I can't close that debt. Because every month I have to buy the groceries for the whole month. So, I'm having a problem as far as the traveling

> expenses are concerned. Particularly if having problems, side effects, or even to go back to collect treatment.

In the face of these difficulties, another woman suggested that the clinic was not sympathetic about money problems. This was contested by the head of the clinic, however, who said they understood these problems and tried to be flexible because they knew patients would eventually come to the clinic, albeit a few days later.

Another group in Stinkwater also talked about their coping strategies, in borrowing money from neighbors to come to the clinic. They cited the role of the disability grant as critical to their ability to repay them. Given the backdrop of economic exclusion and high levels of poverty, the second issue, namely, access to grants, was raised more generally across groups. Several participants were concerned about what would happen to the grant if their health recovered when on treatment. Participants referred to people they knew who, being fearful of losing their disability grant when their CD4 count raises high enough, sought to undermine their recovery: "There're quite a lot of people who don't drink it properly. Then if they don't drink it properly maybe they don't condomize. And if you don't condomize you know that your CD4 count is going to fluctuate. It is going to be 100, still at 100 . . . They take the medication when they are not feeling well and some take the medication everyday but they don't condomize. They don't eat well, or they drink beer, they mix the medication with beer" ("T").

Again, the impact of grants or, more precisely, the fear of losing them, is therefore deterring treatment adherence. But there is also the related concern that, in doing so, because the fear of losing the disability grant as your CD4 count improves encourages some to gamble with their sexual well being and health, is undermining prevention efforts. This is not therefore some irrational or ignorant behavior because respondents tended to know the consequences—in fact, that was the point. Rather, it reflects the economic desperation and grant dependency. The burden of poverty and, hence, the reliance on social grants was also confirmed by a social worker at the clinic who cited lack of income as a big factor in adherence.

The role of government was mentioned in this context. There was a perception that people were deliberately not being encouraged to take ARVs because of the financial implications to government in having to give social grants to patients to obtain food. In other words, some saw this as the reason why government was playing down the benefits of ARVs. A degree of hypocrisy was also mentioned by some of the groups concerning government messages. On the one hand, government told people living with AIDS to eat healthy. But on the other, they are confronted by the daily reality of the difficulty in doing so, particularly when confronting slow and inefficient grant processing. There was the likelihood that, in many cases, patients would die before even receiving the grant. The following exchange captures the bearing socioeconomic hardship has upon attitudes to ARVs:

> *"Thandi":* But then, when your CD4 count rises, they even cut your grant. They say you are strong.
>
> *Facilitator:* If they cut your grant, do you think you still have to take ARVs or just stop taking them?
>
> *"Thandi":* That's why I told you that I have a serious problem with [the Department of] Health and the government because the government they say, 'you should go and work' but they don't give you the job. Where are you going to work?
>
> *"Rose":* "And, because you are still on ARVs, you starve.
>
> *"Thandi":* They used to tell us that once you are positive you need to rest but now they say 'go and work.' But, where and when are you going to rest once you work? *I don't like these ARVs.* I don't like it (emphasis added).

The above conversation reveals a direct link between patient perceptions of ARVs, as seen in earlier chapters, but with the added dimension here of the perceived role of ARVs in socioeconomic well-being. The ARVs were the "reason" someone qualified for a disability grant because it is given related to their stage of illness. But because one's health generally improves on ARVs the grant can be withdrawn due to better health. ARVs may become an indicator of declining economic well-being for some, apparently leading respondents to not like ARVs as a consequence. This may play a role in poorer adherence.

Food was an additional issue identified as a major factor in taking ARVs. In some cases, people talked about patients who sold ARVs in order to get something to eat. The dietician at Wellness, who, in response to being asked if nutrition was a problem confronting patients, also confirmed the problem of inadequate nutrition: "It's a huge problem. Most of them are not working. If they are working it is not a permanent job. Some of them have been cut off from work because they have taken a very long sick leave. They are just on sick leave for, I don't know, a long time. Food security is a huge problem." She estimated that of the ten people she sees daily, nine of them would receive nutritional supplements and that "it is only one out of the ten I see a day that you find they do not need supplements." The head of a home-based care organization, "Minkie," also cited, unprompted, the role of food as the biggest concern for her patients on ARVs. Edgar Makhutle, another key informant, employed by the Moretele District Health Council to trace defaulting patients, said, "if you are hungry I believe that there is nothing that one can do" [i.e., in terms of adherence]. The difficulties associated with ARVs are therefore heightened when, as with cutting the grant, socioeconomic circumstances are poor.

In some cases, the burden of having to find money for transport was eased by treatment, as mentioned, being given by the clinic for longer than one month. In a couple of cases, it is apparently given for three months if the patient can demonstrate that they were adhering well. But returning to the clinic was still a problem for many, and discussion ensued in groups about what people do when they face being without treatment for some days due to inability to get back to the clinic. Some claimed they were suffering and it was encouraging defaulting. Others suggested that Jubilee be informed so that they can give pills to cover days when someone will fall short.

The implication of having to fetch treatment regularly proved to be devastating for one patient. She told of how she had lost her job because of the lack of flexibility in the system for treatment provision and subsequent need for time from work spent queuing. When she inquired about getting treatment for a month she was told: "There is no hospital that will ever give you monthly treatment. I went there to get my treatment every second week. They do not give you any [more] treatment. You have to come back now and then. Imagine if I was working as a domestic worker and had to miss work every Tuesday to come and get the treatment? So I was fired. That is not fair" ("Gloria"). All of this may inhibit people living with AIDS from seeking treatment and, once on it, may discourage them from taking it. Edgar Makhutle suggested that the figure for defaulters at any one time was approximately twenty. This informant suggested that a big factor in defaulting appeared to be a patient's false perception of recovery and may interrupt treatment as a result. Some even regarded themselves as having "healed" completely. Other factors cited were lack of education on ARVs and the problems of side effects. Food, as mentioned, was critical and vegetable gardens were encouraged.

The lack of joined-up thinking in health service provision appears to be a particular characteristic of TB treatment. Because there is a high level of coinfection with HIV/AIDS, TB services are discussed in the following section.

Lack of Flexibility for TB Services

Additional problems include when a patient is traveling and staying in another area. There does not appear to be much flexibility in the system, particularly if a person lacks an appointment, is not registered at that facility, or even if there is an emergency. Respondents described a fragmented TB service, one deemed not to cater to patients.

Unidentified female 1: If you take treatment from the clinic they will not be able to help you unless you ask them to write you a letter referring you to a clinic which is close by your place so that next time you can take your treatment from there. Can I ask a question? I am on the TB treatment and I went to . . . [name of clinic] and the treatment they gave me got finished on Monday and then they told me to go to my clinic and they only gave me three pills and told me to go back to my clinic. I went to my clinic and when I was at the clinic they said I did not make an appointment and then I went another day and they only gave me treatment for one day. I traveled all around getting cold and tired.

Unidentified female 2: I was also on TB treatment in 2003 and I had done it from the other hospital but when I went to another hospital they would not give me unless I go back to the hospital where I went to first, yet I did not have money to go to that clinic because it was far.

Facilitator: Maybe it is because they did not have your record and your record was at the clinic you went to at first?

Female 2: But, what if there is an emergency and I cannot go to the other clinic?

Facilitator: For an emergency they would give you?

Both females at once: They do not give you TB treatment even if it is an emergency. They refuse.

People also have to queue at Jubilee to get treatment. One person claims clinic staff shouted at them because they were at the wrong clinic. But they did not have money to go to the "right" clinic. As a result, that person said that they missed getting treatment, defaulted, and, as a result, had to restart TB treatment in 2004. Rather than always deemed to be the responsibility of the individual, there also appears to be systemic failures that undermine adherence. Yet, we have similarly seen in an earlier chapter (Chapter 4) that nurses can hold particularly judgmental attitudes toward patients who default. But it is lack of flexibility in the system itself, cited here, that appears to exacerbate problems of TB treatment adherence. These reflect structural barriers.

We have looked at a range of socioeconomic barriers. What, then, about clinical criteria and the role they currently play in access to treatment? Indeed, in talking about psycho-social criteria, these are often inherently conditioned by socioeconomic and personal circumstances of patients.

Clinical Criteria and the Role of Psycho-social Factors

In Chapter 2, it was suggested that setting criteria in determining access to ARVs was very significant. It should therefore be important to look at how these issues of criteria-setting affect access in this local community. In particular, questions were posed in order to gauge how Wellness clinic was deviating, or not, in terms of psycho-social factors. Above all, how do patients themselves experience the concrete reality of abstract criteria?

First, one of the most typical issues raised concerned the CD4 count threshold for commencing treatment. Several patients complained about the unreliability of CD4 counts as an indicator of when to commence treatment.[1] Patients claimed that too much emphasis was placed on CD4 counts, which they suggested did not reflect how the patient actually felt or what they were experiencing. One patient recounted how ill his partner had been in spite of having a CD4 count of over 380. Although having AIDS-defining symptoms, she was apparently refused treatment. This appears a particular problem for those having CD4 counts over 200, and was a situation described by some, such as "T," as unfair.[2] It was also claimed that this was impacting socioeconomic well-being by affecting access to grants. Whereas one doctor might use a person's physical appearance to assess eligibility for the disability grant, a social worker may look at the CD4 count. It was claimed that the criteria had shifted from being "stage"-based, initially, to one based exclusively on CD4 count. It is hoped that the revised guidelines for treatment commencement may eliminate some of these problems. But the discrepancies encountered in accessing the disability grant appear to continue.

Treatment Preparation and Criteria: Disclosure

The other significant issue to arise concerning psycho-social criteria concerns that of disclosure in the context of treatment selection and preparation. As the earlier chapter on access criteria suggested, disclosure is specifically stated in the national treatment guidelines as "non-exclusionary" criteria in terms of accessing treatment. That is, health facilities should not use them to exclude people from treatment. However, a brief review of the guidelines indicated that there is a large degree of ambiguity in the guidelines and especially the operational plan. That is, if adherence is an overarching objective, then disclosure may be viewed as a vehicle to achieve that end. The clinic encouraged disclosure but, they stated, without refusing treatment to a patient who did not want to disclose. Indeed, while the medical outcomes are advantageous where a person can disclose, if they do not, the clinic was regarded as having an enlightened head who did not insist upon it as a prerequisite for access.

In terms of the process to access ARVs, prophylaxis, such as Bactrim, is issued as a test for likelihood of adherence and time management. The patients are given on average three sessions of treatment preparation, each of about thirty to forty-five minutes. Usually, according to the social worker, by the second session, they grasp the idea of the importance of adherence. In all, there are nine weeks of preparation, that is, one session every three weeks. In the meantime, the patient also has to complete a form that is used by social workers as the basis for gauging their level of personal attitude and social support. Such questions include when they were tested and found out their status, and whether they have disclosed it, and so on. It was suggested by clinic staff that as much as 25 percent of patients have problems with disclosure. That said, very few, it was claimed, are unable to resolve this. At the time of the interview, the clinic said only five patients had still not disclosed but that they still receive treatment. The social worker underlined that this was not used to exclude patients but it is encouraged. Upon further discussion with both the first and second clinic heads of Wellness, this appears to be an accurate reflection and a position of common understanding amongst Wellness staff. How, then, did patients themselves experience these criteria?

Generally, while most were encouraged to disclose, there was a wide variety of experiences in doing so. For most, the benefits of disclosing were apparent, especially in accompanying or being accompanied by a "buddy":

> Myself, before I took the ARVs, there is someone I went to fetch my medication with. She was positive and I was also positive. She was my "buddy." You know what, when we got there, they picked up people who would be your buddy and we would go for lessons after that they send you to TB. The next day one of the ones who is HIV positive I had accompanied went alone and then they ask her questions. When I arrived at Jubilee I had no trouble, they counseled us and told us about the Bactrim how it works and its side effects and then they gave us Bactrim. We did not go through any trouble. ("Rose")

In the above case, the person not having a buddy appeared to receive additional questions from clinic staff. But there is no evidence of exclusion. Another said: "I was with my mother and I explained to her everything, then I got that support, then I started to . . . join the support group. I was very shy before about what people would say but now I can go and disclose to each and everybody about this disease. I do not have a problem with that" ("Gloria"). So, disclosure and support reflect the ideal of mutual support and, hopefully, that both appear to go hand in hand for adherence. Even when the patient does not disclose, the clinic can make an assessment and the patient may, as suggested, nonetheless receive treatment. "Nonni" suggested that she is able to go alone and get tablets and that she takes this in secrecy, illustrated by her saying "all that is left behind is in the toilet" (in other words, the packaging of the treatment, reflecting the secrecy in taking medication). This was in contrast to another who suggested that this was more the exception than the rule, particularly because they were surprised that someone got treatment when their own family did not know: "Yah, if you do not come with your family they are not going to give you your medication" ("Thandi").

But for some, there is a cost in disclosing that can be an immense burden in seeking treatment. This was duly acknowledged by the head of clinic, who suggested that disclosure did create "domestic" problems for "a minority of patients." Reflecting the emphasis upon disclosure promoted at the clinic, many respondents claim that they were told to disclose, or at least this was their perception. There is inevitably a thin line between encouragement of disclosure and the patient's perception of this as a prerequisite for access. But many patients interpret disclosure as necessary in terms of needing to be accompanied before they could receive ARVs: "They say before they can give me the ARVs I have to come with my mother or friend, someone I can trust"("Violet"). Another claimed that they could not go alone to get medication: "When you go to fetch them and you are alone, they do not give you. You have to go with someone else. The person you share them with. If you go alone, they will not give you. I went alone and they refused to give the ARVs. They told me to come back again and I did yesterday with my brother and they helped me" ("Khumelo"). Another was not asked to bring anyone: "What happened to me, I have seen they ask people, you know, bring somebody, maybe your family to come with you at Wellness maybe for education about ARVs you see, but to me they never said I must come with somebody" ("Thando"). For some, a signed declaration was necessary, adding to difficulties in getting treatment: "I think first time it was difficult—and I had to sign consent forms to start ARVs" (unidentified).

A key informant, a district health promoter, also mentioned the need for a signatory in order for some to get access.[3] But when he conducts home visits to ascertain reasons for a patient abandoning treatment, he claims that often the family does not necessarily know the status of the patient. Often, the patient can be suffering, as they want to tell the family but do not because they are fearful of consequences, such as rejection. Therefore, on one level, it certainly appears that disclosure can be a problematic and painful experience for people living with AIDS that can heighten exclusion and "domestic problems." But on another level, does this necessarily mean that people living with AIDS are actively turned away or forced to disclose? Interviews with clinic staff clearly demonstrate that the clinic does not think so and that they have been cautious in handling this issue. But, nonetheless, people living with AIDS claimed that they had seen others turned away from the hospital because, apparently, "they couldn't answer questions." As the following exchange reveals, it is not uncommon to know of people refused treatment:

"Thandi": We have seen them.
"Thando": There are many of them.
"Sibo": They [the clinic] keep on postponing.

In one case, "Florence" confronted clinic staff to explain why someone she had seen was turned away from the clinic. The response given to her was that they had not adhered to Bactrim. We should remember as well that the majority of these respondents in the focus groups for people living with AIDS are members of either the clinic support group or a support group at the Sunrise Hospice. In other words, most have traveled a considerable distance in their journey dealing with their status, condition, and subsequent treatment. But such patients in support groups should be considered a minority in terms of the overall number of people living with AIDS. To this extent, their awareness of others having problems in the process to access treatment is significant. Overall, focus groups seemed to understand the importance of pill counting and adherence, and also positively linked this to the benefits derived in bringing a family member, or, other person. Some saw disclosure as a choice but that individuals can be told to bring someone with them. But does it, on another level, suggest that people living with AIDS are being burdened with disclosure, being denied treatment, and that this may inhibit them from seeking treatment?

Another respondent said, "they told me that I must bring someone for the first two months. They told us that, I mean the people that I went with they told us that at Wellness that you must bring someone." That disclosure is the preference does not mean the clinic sees it as active exclusion. According to the previous head of the ARV clinic, the emphasis on disclosure merely delays getting treatment.[4] However, for all the rationale of the process, it does appear that people are getting turned away unless they can disclose, at the very least, this slows down access. It may also deter those struggling from returning to the clinic. People living with AIDS also felt that this adherence policy was not consistent across different areas. For example, some claimed that people at other clinics, such as in Mafikeng (in the North West), did not need to drink Bactrim.

There were also differences in opinion concerning the procedure, particularly about whether pills are counted, regarding Bactrim:

"Thandi": What they do is they can count the tablets. They know that they have given you 90 or hundred and something so if you still have them after a week they can see.

> *"Gloria":* You know what, they count the pills that they gave you and they know that they have given you so many pills, so if you throw them away then they know that they had given you so many pills.

This group disagreed and many shouted out that they do not count, while others do. The point seems to be that there are different perceptions and experiences of how the same policy differs in its implementation. It obviously reflects the different circumstances patients find themselves in and the different information or interpretation and understandings of it. But contrary to the claims made by staff that no patient is excluded from treatment, the accounts given by some would appear to suggest otherwise. If not then explicit, the result of the emphasis upon disclosure does appear to have the same result: some patients are filtered out of the process, whether merely delayed or perhaps more permanently. The exclusion, or attrition, rather, lies in the process to initiate treatment itself: "They [the clinic] want a lot from you. They told me to go for a blood test or go open another file. I told them to leave me alone. How could I do that? Now, I'm not taking anything [medication]" ("Thandi"). Perhaps there is therefore a correlation between attrition in the process, mentioned above, and with the same respondent also earlier expressing severe difficulties in terms of grant dependency, transport, financial problems, and lack of social support. This can only lead to the conclusion that while intrinsically reflecting a fair process to access ARVs and, indeed, with the clinic appearing to respond well, some vulnerable patients are excluded or fall off treatment. It is predominantly those with least social support and social and economic problems, which exacerbate their problems in dealing with the treatment initiation procedure.

This may, thankfully, be a small minority of patients. But are they precisely the ones identified by Paul Farmer "who are least likely to comply who are those least likely to comply"? (Farmer 2005). Undoubtedly, against a backdrop of immense operational difficulties, the clinic has performed amazingly in initiating so many so quickly on to ARVs. But is there a danger that those facing particularly difficult social problems are those being sacrificed for the greater good of the process? And, for the majority apparently coping better with ARVs, they are still encountering significant levels of socioeconomic deprivation that continues to be a threat to adherence. These socioeconomic and treatment process issues are therefore piled on top of all of the additional barriers that have been looked at in this book.

CONCLUSION

Toward Treatment, Rights, and Accountability

What, then, do all these barriers confronting AIDS programs and human rights tell us about the place of both in the first decade of the twenty-first century? Perhaps the most important overall observation is that despite the immense problems, the majority of patients are benefiting from treatment. Many have been able to resume work and social roles that were forsaken by illness to restart life. Many, such as "T," have also been empowered through their profound experiences and turned an often-harrowing situation instead into a precious life-sustaining force. Another observation is that the findings reflect a snapshot of ARV rollout at a particularly acute moment in South Africa. It is therefore hoped that many of the more fundamental obstacles having to do with the range of operational and structural issues identified, such as transformation and strengthening of health services, human resources, and sustainable drug supply, will be vigorously responded to by the state and NGOs. Not least, this book has shown the critical need for unambiguous and accessible information is essential to this and other communities. Patients and communities are undoubtedly gradually gaining this and appreciating that there are more positive than negative attributes to ARVs. But the profound need for better information and regulation of alternative products is still a keenly contested issue in South Africa. To date, this is not being sufficiently resolved. Another area concerns the ongoing stigma associated with AIDS, now transferred onto ARVs. Cultural barriers have also been identified but still appear to receive inadequate attention. It is also unclear whether the revised treatment guidelines and policy take into account adequately the more vulnerable and less socially supported people in need of ARVs. Governance of the process is a critical issue and there is evidence to suggest that there is a lack of accountability and transparency in institutions, such as Jubilee hospital.

Above all, the book has shown how the whole issue of ARV access required navigating the dense political fog thrown up by the scourage of AIDS denialism. It is therefore highly appropriate that the timing of the writing of the book's conclusion overlapped with the ousting of Thabo Mbeki from the presidency of South Africa, by his own political party, the African National Congress. It is firmly hoped that at the cigarette-end of the Mbeki era, the embers of denialism will rapidly fade. Another good portent has also been the removal of the health minister, Manto Tshabalala-Msimang, which followed soon after Mbeki's exit. These key political changes will remove the sources of the most damaging manifestations of denialism in policy making and implementation. There are very encouraging signs that a newly emerging consensus on AIDS policy is developing.

But much remains less clear. Does this hope place too much faith in denialism as somehow idiosyncratic to Mbeki and his term in office? While, arguably, this era damaged the national psyche, scuppering coherent and unified responses to AIDS, these attitudes feed into *and* off other complex factors that go into creating layers of personal denialism within communities (Steinberg 2006). And, as the baton of the presidency is snatched from Mbeki and most likely handed to Jacob Zuma, new concerns will be raised. On the one hand, this will involve scrutiny of how the Zuma brand of virility, masculinity, and populism will impact prevention efforts. These are prevention efforts that require urgent rethink and vigorous leadership. Whether Zuma is most appropriate for this task remains an open question. And in terms of treatment, on the other, Zuma's views on traditional treatment, some of which are recorded in this book, may indicate contradictions with use of ARVs. Alternatively, it can also be argued that it is precisely because of the controversies surrounding Zuma that many difficult issues have now been dredged to the surface of national life and debate. Indeed, can those issues associated with Zuma that were publicly acknowledged now provide the entry point for a more open, nuanced and less polarized national discussion? Can a Zuma presidency therefore be an advantageous moment for South Africa to finally grapple with long overdue concerns that resonate across the country? For example, can Zuma's populist approach perhaps be utilized for a more thorough engagement with difficult issues such as masculinity, traditional medicine and interpretation of illness, AIDS and ARVs? This is because the way information is given and received is critical in the context of responding to AIDS. It is bound up with broader issues of advocacy and social mobilization needed to break the wall of personal denialism in South Africa.

The broader lesson is that all of the above, contrary to a noticeable shift in perceived global wisdom concerning the epidemic, do nothing else other than to confirm the continuing relevance of a rights-based approach. But this must be one more nuanced, flexible and better adapted to the treatment era and new ways of linking the public and private spaces of AIDS. In considering the role of rights in treatment programs and responses to the array of barriers to access and adherence, three key areas are discussed here: ensuring that rights are relevant to communities; the need to broaden conceptualization of the right to health, including access to medication; and, broadening advocacy.

Redeeming Relevant Rights

Given the powerful critiques leveled at rights, evident in Chapter 2, and kinds of structural and cultural barriers and negativity toward them identified in Hammanskraal-Temba, are rights at all redeemable? That is, do they, and can they, remain useful for treatment programs, and, more generally, in confronting the challenges of development? These concerns are heightened if the supposed beneficiaries—rights claimants—are themselves alienated from rights or see them as of little relevance for their day-to-day struggles. The poor image of human rights in the case study area can be attributed to a number of factors.

One elementary fact is that most people did not know about rights and there was little knowledge of, or exposure to, the South African bill of rights. Identifying and rectifying gaps in knowledge may be important as well as good business for human rights education and training organizations. But surely the more fundamental challenge, and one consistently raised by respondents, lies in making rights relevant in a context of cultural difference and poverty and high unemployment. In such an environment, it is absolutely essential for people to see the relevance of rights in their everyday existence. A rights-based discourse, so salient in South Africa, appears to accrue, few, if any, tangible benefits to local areas. Notable exceptions do exist, particularly those concerning litigation on socioeconomic rights at a national level. But these are usually legal successes that test the "reasonableness" of government policy but do not necessarily deliver anything to communities (Jones and Stokke 2005). Arguably, the longer rights remain abstract, irrelevant, or threatening to these "local worlds," the greater the chance that constitutional based human rights in South Africa will be increasingly vulnerable to illiberal challenges. And many of those challenges stem from communities turning to diverse practices in attempting to cope with and understand the epidemic.

A related issue concerns whether communities, even if conceptualizing violations as human rights abuses, are then able to enforce rights. Until the creation of a paralegal service, through the Centre for Study of AIDS's *Tswelopele* project, most people were not able to mention one active human rights organization or institution in Hammanskraal-Temba where they could go to seek assistance with their problems. The fact that many people see human rights as a problem, as suggested, rather than as a means of empowerment, is a fundamental contradiction for the rights-based paradigm. Rights urgently need to be made relevant to communities lest we witness the continuing "human rights drift" in responses to AIDS. To reassert the powerful and important role of rights, therefore, two further dimensions are elaborated upon.

Broadening the Right to Health and Access to Medication

One important dimension exists on a conceptual level with operational implications. The human right to health and access to medication must be both aware and flexible enough to embrace the kinds of structures identified in this book. Taking some inspiration from some recent work done by the South African Human Rights Commission,[1] and adding other components, I wish to briefly elaborate on what a right to health, and especially concerning access to ARVs, should also encompass.

First, in terms of "availability," we should be thinking about the components necessary in order to supply a health service. Certainly, while ARVs must be made available, this is also contingent upon funding commitments and the creation of health facilities, infrastructure, and equipment. Strengthening health systems should be an integral dimension of the right to health. Two critical challenges emerging in the treatment era concern, first, the shortages and turnover in health personnel. As told by patients, this can have a dramatic impact upon their well-being. Sufficient numbers of doctors and nurses need to be competently trained and motivated Second, the ongoing efforts to create a cheap and sustainable supply of ARV and other medication, including generic copies remains of utmost concern.

Second, and in relation to issues involved in availability, as mentioned in Chapter 2, neither political nor institutional barriers are explicitly identified in the right to health framework. It would appear critical to inquire into, for example, the nature and quality of management and staff relations. It is also important to ask about intersectoral issues between different layers of decision-making, such as provincial, district levels and health facility management. Following the International Guidelines on HIV and Human Rights, an important additional dimension in providing services should be that they are done in accordance with the principles of transparency, participation, and accountability in decision-making. These principles should be made benchmarks for a rights-based process. However, such a process should also provide concrete mechanisms to channel community participation, debate and consultation. In other words, appropriate institutional structures are required and whose performance should be scrutinized. Third, issues underpinning ability to access ARVs—their accessibility—include physical barriers posed by geography. The ability to meet transport needs would appear critical. There is also the issue of emergency transport (ambulances), which will also be critical for some people living with AIDS in need of medical treatment. Out-of-pocket expenses are other considerations. These include any related user fees for health services. Other issues might include the waiting time involved, which, if long, may deter people from seeking access. The chapter on socio-economic barriers (Chapter 7) also revealed the critical role of nutrition in adherence to ARVs. Hence the benefits to health from social welfare payments, including campaigning for a universal basic income grant, are apparent. Developing more localized service points is critical in overcoming problems of distance and queuing. There is also a critical role for monitoring access and "who" exactly is accessing treatment. Better availability of data and its disaggregation in terms of aspects such as socio-economic status, gender, age, geographic location, children and other vulnerable groups is integral to monitoring disparities in access. Fourth, also in terms of accessibility, access to information is a so-called empowerment right. Its significance lies in informing and raising consciousness among patients as to their rights. The promotion of treatment literacy is key to this, as is the role of language in facilitating communication. Another dimension is the highly influential role of leadership statements and that these conform to appropriate standards reflecting unambiguous statements on treatment.

Fifth, although the importance of acceptability is mentioned in a right to health paradigm, this is generally not elaborated upon. In the context of ARV use, for example, social acceptability requires ways of tackling the stubborn underlying social attitudes and the persistence of stigma identified in the study. WHO-type documents only fleetingly mention some of those judgmental attitudes or social relations. These can exist between the patient and health care workers or within the community surrounding the good or service in question. In a highly stigmatized environment surrounding HIV/AIDS, these attitudes may have a critical bearing upon decisions made by health care workers to initiate patients on treatment and patients to approach clinics. National treatment guidelines are therefore important to establish clarity on access, as well as training of health care workers in using them. While testing is becoming increasingly routinized, and there are many good epidemiological and medical reasons for this, it should still incorporate a basic level of human rights considerations.

Given the high usage of traditional medication and consultation, cultural accessibility and acceptance would appear particularly apposite for consideration in South Africa, as in many other countries. In this, attitudes of health care workers toward traditional medication and, reciprocally, people living with AIDS toward so-called evidence-based health systems would also appear to impact access.[2] Above all, how the cultural context might be better accommodated and integrated into mainstream ARV service provision is a critical issue. For example, how should clinics tackle the large number of patients who mix medication? And do they inadvertently encourage ARV treatment interruption because they tell patients not to mix? How can adherence challenges related to cultural issues, particularly nonbiomedical explanations for illness, be better dealt with, perhaps in the treatment preparation process and even before then? And the issue of regulation of alternative products needs urgent attention to protect vulnerable people from exploitation, which, in the case study area, as elsewhere, is rampant. Some regulation of healers and traditional practitioners is also clearly warranted, especially to protect more vulnerable groups, including children.

Sixth, a related issue in acceptance concerns the quality of the service in question, also related to availability and resourcing of health services. For example, the attitudes of health care workers and the degree of care shown to patients might also be important for structuring access, particularly should the level of care be deemed unacceptable. The relationship between health care workers' employment conditions, availability, and quality issues is therefore an important consideration. To that extent, it is important to explore how human rights can have a constructive role in enabling a common agenda for health providers and patients alike. How can rights be used to help forge mutual interest rather than adversarial ones? Another critical issue within this area of quality is the need for better integration of TB and ARV services.

Seventh, and finally, the issue of redress for violation of some of these aspects of a right to health, particularly mistreatment of people living with AIDS, is critical in expanding access to medication. The need to hold service providers to account highlights the role of building appropriate mechanisms and channels to enable accountability. The global level political liberalization that de Waal (2006) talks about in the context of responses to AIDS appears not only fickle but also unreciprocated at a local level. Access to legal aid is necessary for any violations to be challenged. But it is also important to ask questions about the quality of legal aid, and what it achieves. Another issue is under what circumstances litigation is deemed more appropriate than nonlegal avenues for redress. These dimensions should therefore be read together as an interrelated package creating and sustaining access to services. Availability of ARVs, for example, is clearly of little point if there are no qualified health care workers to administer them. But then, if there are health care workers who feel undervalued, even excluded by management, then this might fuel some of the negative actions and attitudes toward people living with AIDS.

What is attempted here is some elaboration of the right to health framework. While a right to health is a powerful mechanism to lay a claim to access something, access is a composite of a variety of social, cultural, and political dynamics. It therefore becomes self-evident that human rights and development require greater dialogue and embrace. The book has been premised upon the benefits of encouraging such interactions. It is an inescapable truth, however, that animating these (often complex) rights based principles requires particular kinds of social actors. Rights, after all, will not do anything by themselves.

Broadening Advocacy

Several issues highlighted the critical role that exists for community advocacy. This advocacy is necessary to deal with the local hospital, health care workers, the local AIDS council, local authority councilors, and above all, in demands for unambiguous and consistent information. And the regulation of specific harmful cultural practices and alternative medications all require a voice for action. There is an absence of civil society organizations in the area with which to provide a focal point to tackle these issues. But this might, in part, reflect the local political culture, with alternative mechanisms, such as traditional authorities, consulted in preference to other types of organization. How can responses be better rooted locally, to provide the pressure for accountability inimical to better service delivery? And this component requires urgent attention in the form of treatment literacy and health citizenship while presented in a way that can work with parallel systems.

At the time of writing, although changing, there was still little in the way of advocacy initiatives in the case study area. Yet, respondents themselves mentioned a range of issues to do with lack of, or ambiguous, information, corruption in local politics, ongoing problems in keeping privacy and confidentiality, and the need to workshop health care workers on rights. Additional issues identified were the role of AIDS councilors, who were either not HIV-positive or had refused to test or disclose, were deemed inappropriate. There appears to be an abundance of issues to advocate around but there was no local branch of either the TAC or NAPWA (the National Association of People living with AIDS) in Hammanskraal-Temba during fieldwork. The *Tswelopele* project of the Centre for the Study of AIDS, University of Pretoria, is therefore pivotal in providing legal services and local educational workshops to address stigma and discrimination of people living with AIDS. In just a few years, the caseload dealt with by the project paralegals has jumped into the hundreds. It is hoped that, when appropriate, some of these may be pursued by litigation. The clear majority of cases are employment or finance related, which reflect important local level concerns. One project-related spin-off is the facilitation of a partnership of local AIDS-related services to provide a structure from which to educate, advocate, and liaise with service providers. Another is the assistance given to members of both a local hospice and the local clinic support group to set up a people-living-with-AIDS advocacy group. It is fitting that "T" himself became a key actor in the group and is particularly involved in tackling hospital-related issues. *Tswelopele* therefore helps facilitate better coordination of services, training, workshops, and legal assistance, all of which are absolutely critical to protecting the rights of people living with AIDS. *Tswelopele* is building a structure where there had been little formal protection for people living with AIDS in the area. These services and structures are vital in areas like Hammanskraal-Temba, previously underdeveloped and relegated to the semi-urban periphery of South Africa. But beyond this important role, whether they can or should kick-start a deeper level of community involvement is less clear.

In his discussion of the obstacles identified in a treatment program in Mpumalanga, another part of South Africa, Robins (2006:668) concludes: "Were the socio-cultural obstacles in places like Mpumalanga largely due to the absence of the forms of AIDS activism and health citizenship and subjectivities promoted by TAC and MSF? Could TAC and MSF overcome these obstacles to biomedical interventions through their grassroots mobilisation and treatment literacy campaigns?"

The question appears to be equally valid for Hammanskraal-Temba and many other such communities across South Africa. During the study, as mentioned, Hammanskraal-Temba did not have a TAC branch. This has since changed, with a former SANCO activist recently involved in creating a branch. Is one solution, therefore, to have a TAC branch in every community? Although Robbins does not directly provide an answer, no doubt he would, like others, draw attention to the beneficial ways in which TAC activism and health citizenship have brought a critical vibrancy to responses to AIDS. They are also bound up with the personal experiences and biographies of patients in overcoming the immense social exclusion, fear, and anxieties associated with being HIV-positive. There is not the space here to provide an assessment of the TAC but the immense role played by the TAC, documented elsewhere, is acknowledged.

Not least, this form of civil society activism has been integral to challenging government inaction on, and opposition to, treatment. It has done so by building linkages between the lived realities of people living with AIDS in "local world" community settings and scaling these up to the democratic spaces created post-1994. The TAC has been a massive factor in people finding and creating the will and purpose to live with AIDS. That, in itself, should be as much to ask of any organization. But, in addition, in locating itself within South Africa's democratic and human rights "spaces," it has breathed new life into the latter. It has used these spaces, animated them, and made them mean something. Contrary to their critics, and charges that this is merely reformist activity, TAC's performance of citizenship, in the long run, will be absolutely critical to the longevity of South Africa's democracy and human rights edifice.

On a more local level, though, we are still discovering how TAC also encounters problems in tackling those complicated structures surrounding sociocultural belief and local governance issues. TAC experiences at the local level need closer scrutiny before anything definitive can be said about them. But it can be suggested that people living with AIDS in Hammanskraal-Temba perhaps require that critical interface TAC brings in dealing with complicated local politics and AIDS treatment services. Whether the TAC is able, capable, or appropriate in filling this activist vacuum in the area remains to be seen. There are still complex issues about how, for some, its activist style is perceived as inappropriate, even arrogant. The jury is also still out regarding how successfully the TAC is tackling issues so key to treatment adherence and AIDS prevention but so fraught with controversy: traditional belief, women's rights and sexuality, among others. And certainly, there is no single solution. But what is clearer is that getting a successful advocacy formula is an essential step in anchoring the place of rights and treatment in the twenty-first century.

The scale of challenges to human rights and treatment programs is immense. It calls for a multifaceted response. This response is difficult and complex to create. But it is exactly what should underpin human rights approaches if they are to remain relevant to and dynamic in improving treatment and responding to AIDS more generally in the years to come.

Appendix

A Note on Methodology

Four principal methods were undertaken in order to produce empirical and ethnographic evidence from people's lived realities.

The principal method involved five focus groups, four conducted with people living with AIDS (PLWA), and one with people not living with AIDS in the community. A total of around fifty people were involved in these focus groups. A group discussion was also held with people living with AIDS and their home-based care organization (KI 19) and another home-based care organization (KI 20).

The second principal method was interviewing, with a total of twenty-five key informant interviews (all with author, except two from the 2004 work; Zuberi et al 2004). These informants were primarily from the Community Based Organization sector, and institutional actors such as the local ARV clinic, local municipality (particularly Moretele), including the Local AIDS Council, as well as the South African National Civic Organization, Congress of South African Trade Unions, residents, and PLWA.

A third method was the use of a questionnaire in order to get some (albeit qualified) statistical verification from the PLWA support group at the ARV clinic.

A fourth method involved collecting secondary materials and review and analysis of them: from ward-level census information to newspaper articles and academic articles.

All of these methods were underpinned by observation in order to use grounded theory based on accounts conveyed and interpreted at local level. Some of the major confounders and "health" warnings concerning the study are pointed out as follows.

Language use. Most of the focus groups were conducted in a local language to make the discussions more accessible and naturally flowing. Translation of these discussions therefore risks losing some of the accuracy and literal meaning. And literacy was obviously an issue for the questionnaire, with respondents having varying degrees of literacy, and, although the questionnaire was explained in a local dialect, this could not surmount basic literacy issues and misunderstanding of the questions in some cases. Transcribing these discussions into English was yet another sieve of the locally grounded and literal meanings.

There are also specific issues in the South African research setting having to do with race. Not always apparent to the researcher, they were undoubtedly present. But they are part also of more general problems whereby respondents refract responses by what they might think the researcher wanted them to say. Attempts were therefore made to avoid leading questions as much as possible and to verify statements with other sources.

The positionality of the Centre for Study of AIDS' (CSA) Tswelopele project in relation to this research was also a factor. The office manager assisted greatly in organizing focus groups and interviews, which inevitably reflects use of his personal contacts and networks, perhaps to the exclusion of others. But, at the same time, this local facilitator undoubtedly enabled access to a variety of respondents than would have otherwise been the case.

Focus group samples always run the risk of not being representative. And, in addition, dynamics within the groups mean that more dominant people or persons are likely to imprint their views on the group whereas perhaps quieter members are not able to express themselves. This method runs the risk of skewing the group discussion to an artificial consensus on some issues. That said, efforts were made to include all and to pursue dissent and alternative views. The female participants did not appear particularly influenced one way or another by the gender mix in these groups. Ultimately, for all these qualifications, a great deal of information was gathered from group discussions. A critical advantage of this method involves the views and opinions gathered that reflect knowledge created *in situ*, in other words, knowledge as it is most likely to be talked about, constructed, and relayed within a community setting (in contrast, for example, to patient cohorts that dwell on individual perceptions).

Individual interviews were kept as open-ended as possible, but again, were inevitably influenced by the relationship between researcher and interviewee. For all the limitations, they were an important source of information, and issues picked up from the focus group could be triangulated with key informant views and the questionnaire.

Contextual information from secondary sources carries the major "health" warning that the census data used is from 2001, and is therefore considerably out of date in a context of service delivery.

On the issue of people-living-with-AIDS respondents, most of those recruited to focus groups were from support groups either based at the clinic and/or a local hospice. There does remain the issue of people living with AIDS who are either not in such groups and/or were described by participants as "hiding at home." The sample of people living with AIDS is therefore inevitably skewed to those already supported in some way, and thus many of the issues discussed and opinions offered are of people living with AIDS who have, in most cases, come to terms with their status and all that implies in terms of disclosure, acceptance, and adherence. That said, this merely underscores the importance of support-group membership. And, in addition, there are immense difficulties, ethical and otherwise, in attempting to target people who have not tested or disclosed. However, some attempts were made to discuss these issues with home-based carers involved in looking after "hard to reach" people living with AIDS.

Finally, in terms of ethical approach, the research followed the ethical code of conduct that has guided the *Tswelopele* project at CSA, University of Pretoria since it was established. For example, if respondents requested anonymity, this has been granted. And, whether requested or not, respondents were informed about the purpose of the research and what the objectives and end product would be. All names of people-living-with-AIDS respondents have been changed.

List of Interviews and Focus Groups

Interviews

1) Dr. Cameron, Jubilee hospital, KI 1, interview, January 30, 2006.
2) Louise du Plessis, Legal Resource Centre, KI 2, interview, February 7, 2006.
3) Dr. Moshabela, Jubilee/Wellness, KI 3, interview, February 17, 2006.
4) Precious, social worker, Jubilee/Wellness, KI 4, interview, February 28, 2006.
5) Dietician, Jubilee/Wellness, KI 5, interview, February 28, 2006.
6) "T," KI 6, interview, March 28, 2006.
7) Moretele Community Radio DJ, KI 7, interview, April 16, 2006.
8) Minkie, Perseverance Rural Development Centre, KI 8, interview, September 7, 2006.
9) Kenny, Area Coordinator, Local AIDS Council, Moretele, KI 9, interview, November 2, 2006.
10) Edgar Makhutle, Health Promotion, Moretele District Health Council (and nonadherence follow-up for Wellness), KI 10, interview, November 2, 2006.

11 and 12) "X" and "Y," COSATU representatives for Moretele, KI 11 and KI 12, interview, November 5, 2006.

13) Brigitte Schaeffler, long-term resident of Hammanskraal, KI 13, interview, November 19, 2006.
14) Dr. Francois Venter, Head of SA Clinicians society (conducted by Mathew Splitek), KI 14, telephone interview, April 20, 2006.

15) Dr. Maharaj, CSIR, Bioscience Unit, KI 15, interview, November 26, 2006.
16) SANCO activist/Hammanskraal, anonymous, KI 16, interview, November 27, 2006.
17) Dr. Mathibedi, Head of Wellness ARV clinic, KI 17, interview, November 27, 2006.
18) Able, Head of Communications, Moretele Local Municipality, KI 18, interview, November 27, 2006.
19) Anonymous home-based care and people living with AIDS, Stinkwater, K19, interview/observation, February 27, 2007.
20) Perseverance Rural Development Centre, K20, interview, April 8, 2007.
21) SANCO Activist/Hammanskraal, anonymous, K16, second interview, May 7, 2007.
22) Martha Ntobeng, former resident, 24 Block B, Temba, KI 21, interview, May 31, 2007.

Plus, from 2004 Tswelopele Research archive:

23) Chief Nawa (classified as KI 17, March 2, 2004).
24) Traditional healers (anonymous) (classified as KI 19, May 11, 2004).
25) Gertrude, social worker (classified as KI 21, May 13, 2004).

Focus Groups

1) People living with AIDS FG 1, Sunrise hospice (twenty-four people: twelve men, twelve women), March 16, 2006.
2) People living with AIDS FG 2, Jubilee support group (seven people: five women and two men), July 24, 2006.
3) People living with AIDS FG 3 (four people: three women, plus "T"), also members of Jubilee group, July 31, 2006.
4) Not people living with AIDS FG 4 (eight people: two men, six women), August 29, 2006.
5) People living with AIDS FG5, mixed, not just Jubilee or Hammanskraal (eight people: seven women and one man), August 29, 2006.

Questionnaire Information

Based on a questionnaire, given in English and Setswana, to people living with AIDS who are in the Jubilee Support Group:

Respondent No.	*M/F*	*Age*	*Ward*	*On ARVs Y/N*	*Wellness Y/N*	*Traditional medication Y/N*	*Positive or negative about taking ARVs?*
1	F	30	Kiogogelo	Y	Y	N	-
2	F	29	73/Hk	Y	Y	N	-
3	F	27	74/5/Tba	Y	Y	N	P
4	F	28	NW/ Makapanstad	Y	Y	N	P
5	F	39	75/5/Tba	Y	Y	-	P
6	F	25	73/Hk	Y	Y	-	P
7	F	31	73/Ramotse	Y	Y	N	P
8	F	34	73/Ramotse	Y	Y	-	-
9	F	31	75	Y	Y	-	P
10	F	47	NW/ Makapanstad	Y	Y	-	-
11	F	33	75/Leboneng	Y	Y	-	P
12	F	40	74/5/Tba	N	N	-	Negative
13	M	55	73/Hk	N	N	-	P
14	M	40	8/Suurman	Y	N	-	P
15	F	47	74/5/Temba	Y	Y	Tradit. Can't heal as not accurate	P
16	M	36	NW/ Makapanstad	Y	Y	-	both
17	F	30	Soshanguve	N	N	-	P although scared of toxicity
18	F	55	14/ Stinkwater	N	N	-	P
19	M	36	74/Kanana	Y	Y	-	-
20	F	42	74/Eersterus	-	-		

Findings

Respondent	*Knowledge on ARVs*	*How easy is it to get ARVs (A-E)?*	*Most important issues in access*	*Groups finding it hardest*	*Adherence Problems*	*Problems of ARVs*	*Additional suggestions*
1	Y	A	Viral information given on role of treatment	Many people	Need food is biggest challenge	-	Talk to health staff
2	Y	A	Get ready, Be determined, stay healthy/personal preparation	No one	Need to take on time	Side effects	Know CD4 count Ask question to understand
3	Y	A	No money. Lack of support at home	Those not disclosing or accepting status	Not adhering. Not disclosing. Stigma. Lack of acceptance	Adherence	Support groups
4	Some	A	-	No one	Vomiting, getting tired	-	-
5	N	B	Test and CD4 count	Myself	No problems taking on time	-	-
6	Y	C	Must go to clinic, check dates of visit, adherence, problems when visiting elsewhere, avoid personal problems	Not following "rules" of hospital, etc.	Viral/personal information		
/attitude	-	Bring treatment supporter to clinic					
7	-	B	Time, reminder, when one lives alone- difficult, when no money for transport to pick ARVs up, it is not possible to have them delivered to you	-	To forget treatment when traveling, drink, smoking	-	-

8	Y	A	Reduced number of people dying, prevent other diseases, need for information	Those not testing	Most relevant-time "not to eat," toxicity	-	Treatment budder/ reminder
9	Y	-	CD4 count, eating healthy, i.e., knowledge	No one	-	-	-
10	Y	C	N	Not hard.	Time, important to eat before take, access to clean water, exercise and vegetables.	It is a right	
11	Y	E	Time, and fear of side effects, have enough sleep, etc.-	School children	-	-	Delivery to (local) clinics
12	Y	A	Knowledge-related	People in rural areas	Knowledge-related	Treatment must be taken to clinics where people are far away from hospitals	
13	"live longer"	B	Knowledge-plus, "to encourage people to have hope of being healed"	Those in denial	Adherence, i.e., forgetting,	Ignorance in obtaining treatment	More (ARV) centers for health established
14	Y	E	Getting grant for life, ARV to nearest clinics. Give to those over 200 Hospital keep those until recover	They fear ARVs			

Respondent	*Knowledge on ARVs*	*How easy is it to get ARVs (A-E)?*	*Most important issues in access*	*Groups finding it hardest*	*Adherence Problems*	*Problems of ARVs*	*Additional suggestions*
15	Yes	E	Money, food, health workers must access people, people rejected	People in villages, impoverished, destitute	Personal knowledge/ attitude. And do many "if."	-	Health workers must go out to people
16	Yes	E	Viral knowledge	Those not knowing status	Poverty, traveling (23ks) to Wellness, ARVs on empty stomach	Social security, when don't have money for travel	
.	-	Social security rights					
17	Yes	C	Money to get to ARV center, counseling and tests- lots, for life time, stigma, food	unemployed	When you feel healthy, timing	-	Every clinic should be a site, and easier options- syrup or treatment breaks
18	Some/yes	B	Viral info.	None	Viral info- side effects and blindness at times	-	-
19	Some/yes	B	Testing (know status), adherence, attendance	The poor	Regular check-ups, high cost of transport, high cost healthy food, not getting enough support from family, life time	-	To have ARVs at local clinics, improve service, i.e., waiting time
20	-	A	Much easier when have transport money	-	Must take them properly	-	-

Notes

Introduction

1. Throughout sub-Saharan Africa, this was well under 1 percent coverage of those needing treatment in 2001, and still only 2 percent in 2004, rising to 28 percent, or 1.3 million people, in 2007, and estimated to have risen, as mentioned, to over 2 million at the end of 2007. See "Toward Universal Access: Progress Report," WHO/UNAIDS (2007, 2008).
2. For "local standards of care" justifications, see Farmer's critique (2005:196–201) in *Pathologies of Power*. See also Jones (2004).
3. In the UNDP report, for example, Botswana had a life expectancy of just 40.3 years by 2000 (UNDP, 2002), which has recently gone down to approximately 39 years, whereas between 1970–75 it was estimated at 53.2 years. Zambia, Uganda, Rwanda, Malawi, Mozambique, Namibia, and Zimbabwe all have lower life expectancy now than over twenty years ago. Most tellingly, for the region as a whole, life expectancy at birth in 1970–1975 was 45.3 years, but by 1995–2000, this had risen to only 48.8 years. This is in marked contrast to much higher overall levels and bigger increases in all other regions except Central and Eastern Europe and the Commonwealth of Independent States (CIS).
4. To illustrate the huge change in ARV prices, Zackie Achmat, then national chairperson of TAC, put this as follows: "Today, the ARV medicines I take cost me R400.00 per month through the private sector. When TAC and our allies started our campaign to reduce the cost of medicine, the same medicine cost at least R4 500.00 per month," "Affidavit," Treatment Action Campaign, available at www.tac.org.za/Documents/Court_Cases/Rath/Defamation/TAC-Achmat-1.pdf, accessed, 06.06.2007.). And see Heywood (2002) for an important account of global mobilization to lower prices.
5. All figures in this section are estimates made by UNAIDS, Global Report (2006).
6. Jones (2004b), for example, looks at PEPFAR and religion, the notion of "partnership" in British AIDS aid.
7. Global HIV Prevention Working Group 'Announcement' (u.d) http://www.gatesfoundation.org/GlobalHealth/Pri_Diseases/HIVAIDS/Announcements/Announce-040610.htm (accessed June 6, 2007).
8. See, for example, Gruskin et al. (2007).
9. Focus Group 2 (see Appendix for details).
10. See "Roundtable on Scaling up HIV Testing," Special Focus (2005), *Health and Human Rights*.

11. Catherine Sozi, UNAIDS country representative, Zambia, interview, Lusaka, in Jones (2007).
12. See Imrie et al (2007) and de Waal (2006), who fear that treatment is the new modus operandi to manage the epidemic.
13. Sozi, in Jones (2007).
14. See Farmer, *Pathologies of Power*, 165.
15. Ibid.
16. The latter point refers to Brazil, in Biehl (2007:67).
17. See, for example, Jones and Stokke (2005); Harriss et al. (2004).
18. Interview, in Jones (2007).
19. Executive Secretary, BONASO, interview, quoted in Jones (2007).
20. See BONELA and Avalos, respectively, in Jones (2007).
21. Dr. Mathibedi, interview, Head of Wellness clinic, Temba (see Appendix for details).
22. These terms and figures are taken from Rosen et al (2007).
23. Sibongile, Khabzela's fiancée, in McGregor (2005:191).

Chapter 1

1. Plusnews (2005) "South Africa: Rollout bogs down," http://www.plusnews.org (accessed, June 10, 2006).
2. This is also echoed in the work of Jonny Steinberg (2006).
3. See for example, Nobel peace laureate claims HIV deliberately created (2004), http://www.abc.net.au/news/newsitems/200410/s1216687.htm (accessed January 15, 2005).
4. This was a project to develop a product that was claimed to be a successful treatment for AIDS. It was subsequently thoroughly discredited and, amongst other things, was found to contain a deadly industrial solvent.
5. See, for example, Kalipeni, Craddock, Oppong, and Ghosh (eds.) (2004).
6. This section draws on Jones (2005a).
7. Mokaba, in *The Sunday Independent*, June 16, 2002.
8. According to William Gumede (2005), Mbeki was apparently incensed a few years earlier at the nature of the Clinton administration's AIDS funding to South Africa which was tied to purchase of branded drugs. This probably contributed to the emphasis given to "underdevelopment" discourse in the Castro Hlongwane document
9. Mokaba, in *The Sunday Independent*, June 16, 2002.
10. See various, such as, De Waal (2003); Mattes (2003), HEARD (2003).
11. See, for example, Patterson (2006); Jones (2005); Friedman and Mottiar (2004); Heywood (2005); Parkhurst and Lush (2004); Putzel (2003a, 2003b); Parkhurst (2001, 2002).
12. The AIDS Program Effort is a useful measurement of AIDS policy responsiveness, as based on USAID, UNAIDS, WHO, and the POLICY Project definitions (in Patterson, 2006: 24–25).
13. The sectors represented within SANAC at this time included: government; parliament; business; people living with AIDS; NGOs; faith-based organizations; trade

unions; women; youth; traditional leaders; legal and human rights groups; disabled people; celebrities; sporting bodies; local government; and the hospitality industry.

14. See Mbeki (2004) in ANC Today.
15. The State and Jacob Zuma (2006).
16. Complainant in the Jacob Zuma "rape" trial testimony, *Pretoria News*, March 7, 2006.
17. "Eat garlic, beetroot and lemon Manto repeats," http://www.iol.co.za/index, June 2006.
18. South African National Department of Health (2004) "HIV and AIDS and treatment," Khomanani, 1st ed., 2004.
19. See, for example, the *Sun* classifieds, February 1, 2007, which lists nine herbalists and their different methods and powers.
20. TAC press release, August 15, 2006. See http://www.tac.org.za.
21. "Time to sack health minister," *Sunday Times*, August 20, 2006.
22. *Pretoria News*, January 12, 2006.
23. Quoted in Fakir (2007:9).
24. "Instability will spread until the state gets its act together," *Sunday Times*, July 11, 2007.
25. "The awful state of the nation," *Mail and Guardian*, October 28, 2005. In many ways, these developmens are a vindication of William Gumede's thesis (2005).
26. See, for example, http://www.pambazuka.org/en/category/rights/32594.
27. A Human Rights Watch researcher said: "It's a shocking irony that people demonstrating for essential medicines should be met with rubber bullets and teargas . . . South Africa should be easing the suffering of people with AIDS, not violently dispersing peaceful demonstrations" (See, Human Rights Watch, 2005).
28. Even when this requirement is met, the magistrate's court rules can be used to interpret the act in a way that make it easier to prohibit gatherings. A civil liability clause for damages also heightens tensions. More troublesome, when acting in bad faith, there appears to be use of this act to augment growing intolerance of police to poor communities' right to demonstrate. This intolerance is also instigated by local authorities invoking the *Regulation of Gatherings Act*, including its apparent misuse—e.g., not responding within twenty-four hours to a properly filed notice, and spurious grounds for prohibition (such as disruptions to traffic, and reasonable suspicion of lawlessness rather than the act's requirement of "credible information on oath," etc) in order to prevent demonstrations. See, for example, Currie and de Waal, J. (2006).
29. See, for example, the speech by the deputy president on the occasion of the keynote address to the National Conference to finalize the national strategic plan on HIV and AIDS, 2007–2011.
30. 'Frere "A national emergency,"' *Daily Dispatch*, http://www.dispatch.co.za/specialreports/article.aspx?id=167088.
31. See, for example, "Letter from the president," http://www.anc.org.za/ancdocs/anctoday/2007/at29.htm.

Chapter 2

1. See Article 12 2c, International covenant on economic social and cultural rights (1966); committee on economic, social and cultural rights (2000); UN CESCR general comment 14 (2000).
2. See, for example, the wide-ranging collection of papers edited by Andreassen and Marks (2006) that take an exemplary multidisciplinary approach to the topic.
3. Gready and Ensor (2005) provide a useful summary.
4. See both Gready and Ensor (2005)and Archbold (2003).
5. See WHO (2003b:6).
6. See, for example, Khoza (2007).
7. South African bill of rights, constitution of the republic of South Africa, Act 108 of 1996, Chapter 2.
8. UN General Assembly, 59th sess. (2005).
9. UNAIDS' HIV/AIDS and human rights international guidelines, revised guideline number 6 (1996, 2002).
10. A very important corrective has been Ruth Macklin's work in particular at the WHO, see later section.
11. See Plusnews (2005) "Lazarus drug: ARVs in the treatment era http://www.irinnews.org (accessed September 10, 2005).
12. See, for example, Report from Malawi, "Equity and the expansion of access to treatment and care in Southern Africa," Equinet workshop, 13th ICASA conference, 2003, Nairobi.
13. According to Norwegian Ministry of Foreign Affairs (2002:33, 36).
14. K. Y. Amoako, Chairman of the Commission on HIV and Governance in Africa, *AIDS Policy Africa*, 1 (1) March, 2004.
15. My thanks to Mathew Splitak for his assistance in doing background research for this section.
16. See UNAIDS (1996) guideline 1.
17. Such as UNAIDS (2003).
18. Question by author to Dr. Simelela on occasion of presentation of the Operational Plan, 27.2.2004, Centre for Study of AIDS, AIDS Forum, University of Pretoria seminar.
19. Telephone interview, April 20 2006.
20. When Dr. Venter spoke of WHO policy, he was likely thinking of WHO's clinical guidelines, the first version of which was published in 2002, and not of the ethical guidelines, which did not appear until 2004.
21. South Africa National Department of Health (2004).
22. See http://www.tac.org.za/community/files/DraftDoHGuidelinesManagementOfHIV2008.doc#_Toc194192429, draft 3.
23. See Joint Civil Society Monitoring Forum website, www.JCSMF.org.za.
24. Following section refers to the South Africa National Department of Health (2004).
25. Person living with HIV/AIDS, discussion at Access to Legal Services Conference, AIDS Law Project, February 2006.
26. The following section refers to the South Africa National Department of Health "Care Plan" (2003).

27. Worries of patient non-adherence could, for example, cause a government to prefer a lead regimen of ARVs packaged in simple fixed-dose combinations or blister packs (15) or a pediatrician to prescribe treatment amenable to coordination with treatment given to a patient's HIV-positive parent.

Chapter 3

1. "ABSA Chain: Henk Rossouw in conversation with Bongani Madondo," https://www.givengain.com/cgi-bin/giga.cgi?cmd=cause_dir_news_item&cause_id=1270&news_id=2916&cat_id=178 (Accessed, November 20 2006).
2. For a review of the "implosion" debate, see the collection in Southall, Segar, and Donaldson (eds.) (1992) and Peires (1992). The failure of ethnic nationalism is described in Bank (1995).
3. SANCO leader, Hammanskraal, interview, KI 16 (See Appendix for this and all interviews).
4. M. Ntobeng, KI 22, interview.
5. M. Ntobeng, KI 22, interview.
6. See also van Huyssteen (2000).
7. City of Tshwane (2005)Integrated Development Plan, p. 29., Pretoria.
8. Ibid.
9. See, "Integrated Development Plan Needs," http://www.tshwane.gov.za/idpneeds/ (accesssed, October 15 2006).
10. Resident, quoted in "Imbizo get an earful of Temba woes," *North West Mirror*, January, 2005.
11. *Pretoria News*, "No new buildings for 'school of shame,'" January 11, 2007.
12. Interviews KI 11 and 12.
13. Interview KI 20.
14. The Offical Ward Based needs Register of the previous 5-year IDP cycle, Zone a, Ward 75, see note 14.
15. However, as of 2007, a major step toward more inclusive and functional boundaries lies in the wards under City of Tshwane being incorporated into the Gauteng province, e.g., twenty-two schools were to be handed over to Gauteng from North West, January 15, 2007, *Pretoria News*, January 8.
16. See http://www.elections.org.za/.
17. SANCO activist, KI 16, interview.
18. Ibid.
19. KI 22, interview.
20. See KI 19.
21. KI 13.
22. The author attempted, several times, to secure an interview with local councillors but to no avail.
23. Chief Nawa, interview, May 11, 2004, Tswelopele documents, KI 19, csa.org.za.
24. SANCO informant in Zuberi et al. (2004).
25. Gertrude, Social Worker, May 13, 2004, Tswelopele documents, KI 21, www.csa.org.za.
26. SANCO respondent, KI 16.

27. See Open Democracy Advice Centre Annual Report (2005:3) at http://www.opendemocracy.org.za/documents/AnnualReport2005.doc.
28. "Mayor slammed for abuse of power," *Citizen*, February 28, 2007.
29. "Residents riot over poor service delivery," *Pretoria News*, April 11, 2007.
30. Resident quoted in "Imbizo get an earful of Temba woes," *North West Mirror*, January, 2005.
31. See http://www.int.iol.co.za/index.php?set_id=1&click_id=594&art_id=nw20070801143735693C611698.

Chapter 4

1. KI 11 and 12.
2. Ntobeng, interview, KI 22.
3. Male person living with AIDS, in Zuberi et al (2004).
4. KI 5.
5. See von Holdt and Murphy (2007) and Schneider et al (2007).
6. Ibid.
7. KI 11 and 12.
8. KI 1, Dr. Cameron.
9. KI6, SANCO activist and KI 22, Ntobeng.
10. KI 6, "T."
11. KI 2.
12. K17, Dr. Mathibedi.
13. KI 14.
14. KI 4.

Chapter 5

1. This Chapter draws heavily on the range of focus group discussions recorded in the Appendix, questionnaire data, also in the Appendix, as well as several key informant interviews.
2. KI 17.
3. KI 3
4. KI 5.
5. KI 6.
6. KI 8.
7. KI 4.

Chapter 6

1. Berger and Heywood also mention a WHO definition of traditional medicine as: ". . . diverse health practices, approaches, knowledge and beliefs incorporating plant, animal and/or mineral based medicines, spiritual therapies, manual techniques and exercises applied singularly or in combination to maintain well-being, as well as to treat, diagnose or prevent illness."
2. *Muti* is a play on the name for traditional healer medicine.

3. Ibid., p. 536.
4. Of course, this has gained momentum with, for example, the creation of an expert Committee on African Traditional Medicine and, as mentioned, involvement of the CSIR, MRC, and Department of Health in collating a database of plant related medications (see Berger and Heywood, 2007).
5. As one example, some deemed that it should not be used by pregnant women because it may be harmful.
6. Another example was of something called *Subhukulu*, mentioned as beneficial and only problematic with incorrect usage.
7. In Zuberi et al. (2004) it was not attempted to unpack the concept and practice of witchcraft, which was lumped together with Makhome.
8. KI 8.
9. Zuberi et al. (2004); plus, author's field notes, and Tswelopele project documents, KI 17, March 2, 2004 available at http://www.csa.org.za.

Chapter 7

1. This chapter draws heavily upon focus group material in particular (for more information on these, see Appendix).
2. KI 6.
3. KI 10.
4. KI 3.

Chapter 8

1. This was one of many interesting points, some reflected in this section, to come out of Ntuli's (n.d.) report on behalf of the South African Human Rights Commission (SAHRC).
2. SAHRC (undated).

Bibliography

ABSA Chain. (n.d.). Henk Rossouw in conversation with Bongani Madondo, http://www.givengain.com/cgi-bin/giga.cgi?cmd=cause_dir_news_item&cause_id=1270&news_id=2916&cat_id=178 (accessed November 20, 2006).

A'desky, A. (2004). *Moving mountains: The race to treat global AIDS*. Verso Books.

AIDS Law Project (2008), "Joint submission on the draft medicines and related substances amendment bill," http://www.tac.org.za/community/files/SubmissionOnMedicinesActBill-20080515.pdf (accessed June 1, 2008).

AIDS and Rights Alliance for Southern Africa. (2006). *HIV/AIDS and human rights in SADC*. Windhoek.

African National Congress. (2004). Nevirapine, drugs and African guinea pigs. *ANC Today, 4(40)*, http://www.anc.org.za/ancdocs/anctoday/2004/at50.htm (accessed February 2, 2005).

Andreassen, B. A., & Marks, S. P. (2006). *Development as a human right*. Harvard School of Public Health.

Archibold, C. (2003). The incorporation of civic and social rights in domestic law. In J. Coicaud et al (Eds.), *The globalization of human rights* (pp. 56–86). United Nations University Press.

Ashforth, A. (2000). *Madumo: A man bewitched*. University of Chicago Press.

Atkinson, D. (2007). Taking to the streets. Has developmental local government failed in South Africa? In Buhlungu, S., Daniel, J., Southall, S., and Lutchman, J. (Eds.), *State of the nation* (pp. 53–77).

Bank, L. (1995). The failure of ethnic nationalism: Land, power, and the politics of clanship on the South African highveld. *Africa, 65*(4).

Berger, J., Hassim, A. and Heywood, H. (2007). 'Traditional and Alternative Health Care' in Berger et al (2007). *Health and Democracy*, pp. 200–225. Siber Ink.

Biehl, J. (2007). *Will to live: AIDS therapies and the politics of survival*. Princeton University Press.

Booysen, F., Anderson, S., & Meyer, K. (2006). Public sector antiretroviral treatment: The challenge of patient retention. *Acta Academica Supplementum, 1*, 309–38. University of the Free State.

Buhlungu, S., Daniel, J., Southall, S., & Lutchman, J. (Eds.). (2007). *State of the nation: South Africa 2007*. Pretoria: HSRC Press.

Cameron, E. (2000). The deafening silence of AIDS. *Health and Human Rights 2000, 5*(1), 7–24.

———. (2005). *Witness to AIDS*. I. B. Tauris.

Campbell, C. (2003). *Letting them die: Why AIDS intervention programmes fail.* James Currey.

Chopra, M., Kendall, C., Hill, Z., Schaay, N., Nkonki, L. L., & Doherty, T. (2006). "Nothing new": Responses to the introduction of antiretroviral drugs in South Africa. *AIDS, 20,* 1975–1977.

City of Tshwane. (2005). Integrated Development Plan, http://tshwane.gov.za (accessed January 12, 2006).

———. (2006). Integrated Development Plan Needs Register, http://www.tshwane.gov.za/idpneeds/ (accessed October 15, 2006).

Constitution of the Republic of South Africa. (1996). Act 108 of 1996, Chapter 2, Bill of Rights.

Complainant in the Jacob Zuma "rape" trial testimony. (2006). *Pretoria News,* March 7.

Craddock, S. (2000). *City of plagues: Disease, poverty and deviance in San Francisco.* University of Minnesota Press.

Currie, I., & de Waal, J. (2006). *The bill of rights handbook.* Juta Publishers.

Daniels, N. (2004). How to achieve fair distribution of ARTs in 3 by 5: Fair process and legitimacy in patient selection. Geneva: WHO.

de Waal, A. (2003). How will HIV/AIDS transform African governance? *African Affairs, 102,* 1–23.

———. (2006). *AIDS and power.* Zed Books.

"Eat garlic, beetroot and lemon Manto repeats," (2006). http://www.iol.co.za/index, June (accessed July 10 2006).

Eide, A. (2003). Making human rights universal in an age of economic globalisation. In S. von Schlorlemer (Ed.), *Praxis-handbuch UNO: Die Vereinten Nationen im Lichte globaler Herausforderungen* (pp. 241–62). Springer.

Englund, H. (2006). *Prisoners of freedom: Human rights and the African poor.* University of California Press.

Evans, T. (2002). A human right to health? *Third World Quarterly, 23*(2), 197–215.

Fakir, E. (2007). Public service delivery in a democratic developmental state. *Policy Issues and Actors, 20*(3).

Farmer, P. (2005). *Pathologies of power: Health, human rights and the new war on the poor.* University of California Press.

Fassin, D. (2007). *When bodies remember: Experiences and politics of AIDS in South Africa.* University of California Press.

Ferguson, J. (1992). *The anti-politics machine: "Development," depoliticization, and bureaucratic power in Lesotho.* University of Minnesota Press.

Fox, R., C. & Goemaere, E. (2006). They call it "patient selection." In Khayelitsha: The experience of Médecins Sans Frontières-South Africa in enrolling patients to receive antiretroviral treatment for HIV/AIDS. *Cambridge Quarterly Healthcare Ethics, 15,* 302–12.

Frere: A national emergency. (2008). *Daily Dispatch,* http://www.dispatch.co.za/special reports/article.aspx?id=167088 (accessed May 13, 2008).

Friedman, S. (2006). Participatory governance and citizens action in post-apartheid South Africa. International Institute for Labour Studies, Decent Work programme (DP/164/2006), Geneva.

Friedman, S., & Mottiar, S. (2004). A rewarding engagement? The treatment action Campaign and the politics of AIDS. Centre for Civil Society Working Paper, University of KwaZulu-Natal.

Global HIV Prevention Working Group "Announcement" (n.d.). http://www.gatesfoundation.org/GlobalHealth/Pri_Diseases/HIVAIDS/Announcements/Announce-040610.htm (accessed June 6, 2007).

Golooba-Mutebi, F., & Tollman, S. (2007). Confronting HIV/AIDS in a South African village: The impact of health-seeking behaviour. *Scandinavian Journal of Public Health, 35*(3), 175–80.

Gready, P., & Ensor, J. (2005). *Reinventing development: Translating rights based approaches from theory into practice*. Zed Books.

Greenstein, R. (2003). State, civil society and the reconfiguration of power in post-apartheid South Africa. Centre for Civil Society, University of KwaZulu Natal.

Gruskin, S., Ferguson, L., & Bogecho, D. (2007). Beyond the numbers: Using rights-based perspectives to enhance antiretroviral treatment scale-up. *AIDS, 21*(5), 13–19.

Gumede, W. (2005). *Thabo Mbeki and the battle for the soul of the ANC*. Zebra Books.

Harriss, J., Stokke, K., & Törnquist, O. (2004). *Politicising democracy: The new local politics of democratisation*. Palgrave-Macmillan.

Hassim, A., Heywood, M., & Berger, J. (2007). *Health and democracy*. Cape Town: Siber Ink.

Health and Human Rights. (2005). Roundtable on scaling up HIV testing. Special focus: Emerging issues in HIV/AIDS. *Health and Human Rights, 8*(2).

HEARD. (2003). *Workshop on HIV/AIDS, democracy and development in South Africa*. Durban, Health Economics and HIV/AIDS Research Division (HEARD).

Hellum, A. (1999). *Women's human rights and legal pluralism in Africa: Mixed norms and identities in infertility management in Africa*. Tano-Aschehoug.

Heywood, M. (n.d.). HIV and AIDS: From the perspective of human rights and legal protection. In *One step further—responses to HIV/AIDS* (pp. 11–28). SIDA studies, SIDA, Art. Nr. SIDA 1693en.

———. (2002). Drug access, patents and global health: "Chaffed and waxed sufficient." *Third World Quarterly, 23*(2), 217–31.

———. (2003). The silence of the lions The HIV/AIDS epidemic and dual loyalties in the New South Africa. Presentation, 2nd Harold Wolpe lecture of 2003, University of Kwazulu-Natal.

———. (2004). (Ed.). From disaster to development? HIV and AIDS in southern Africa. *Development Update, 5*(2).

———. (2005). Shaping, making and breaking the law in the campaign for a national HIV/AIDS treatment plan. In P. Jones & K. Stokke (Eds.) *Democratising Development: The Politics of Socio-Economic Rights in South Africa*. Martinus Njihoff.(pp. 181–212).

Human Rights Watch. (2005). South Africa: Police fire on peaceful AIDS protestors http://www.hrw.org/english/docs/2005/07/13/safric11326.htm (accessed August 2005).

Høg, E. (2006). Human rights and access to AIDS treatment in Mozambique. *African Journal of AIDS Research, 5*(1), 49–60.

Ignatieff, M. (2001). *Human Rights as politics and idolatry*. Princeton University Press.

Imrie, J., Elford, J,. Kippax, S., and Hart, G. (2007). BioMedical HIV Prevention and Social Science. *Lancet*, 370, pp. 10–11.

"Instability will spread until the state gets its act together," (2007). *Sunday Times*, July 11.

International HIV/AIDS Alliance. (2002). Voices from the community—A report of a community consultation on antiretroviral treatment in Zambia.

Jarosz, L. (1992). Constructing the dark continent: Metaphor as geographic representation. *Geogfiska Annaler, 74B*, 105–14.

Joint Civil Society Monitoring Forum (2005). Report, http://www.jcsmf.org.za/?q=node/40/print (accessed June 10, 2006).

Jones, P. S. (1999). From nation-hood to regionalism to the North West province: Bophuthatswananess and the birth of the New South Africa. *African Affairs, 98*, 509–34.

———. (2004a). When "development" devastates: Donor discourses, access to HIV/AIDS treatment in Africa and rethinking landscapes of development. *Third World Quarterly, 25*(2), 385–404.

Jones, P. S. (2004b). Of Gifts and Return Gifts: Beyond the political and practical deficits of donor assistance. *Development Update*, 5 (3), 157–82.

———. (2005a). "A test of governance": Rights-based struggles and the politics of HIV/AIDS policy in South Africa. *Political Geography, 2* (4), 419–47.

———. (2005b). "On a never ending waiting list": Towards equitable access to antiretroviral treatment? Experiences from Zambia. *Health and Human Rights, 8*(2).

———. (2007). Beyond barriers: Towards extending AIDS medication in Southern Africa. Report to OSISA. Centre for the Study of AIDS, University of Pretoria.

Jones, P. S., & Koffeld, K. (2008). Governance matters for AIDS: But what about the politics? Lessons from South Africa and Uganda. In M. Foller & H. Thörn (Eds.), *The Politics of AIDS: Globalization, the state and civil society* (pp. 97–122). Palgrave Macmillan.

Jones, P. S., & Stokke, K. (Eds.). (2005). *Democratising development: The politics of socio-economic rights in South Africa*. Martinus Nijhoff.

Jonsson, U. (2005). A human rights based approach to programming. In Gready and Ensor (Eds.). pp. 47–62.

Justice Africa (2007). GAIN Issues Brief No. 10, "Global Health Roundtable."

Kalipeni, E., Craddock, S., Oppong, J. R., & Ghosh, J. (Eds.). (2004). *HIV and AIDS in Africa: Beyond epidemiology*. Blackwell Publishing.

Karim, A. S. S., & Karim, A. Q. (2005). *HIV/AIDS in South Africa*. Cambridge University Press.

Kårsholm, P. (2006). Culture as cure: Civil society and moral debates in Kwa-Zulu Natal after apartheid. In P. Kåarsholm & I. Hofmeyr (Eds.), Popular Cultural Materials and Public Sphere, *Current Writing, 18*(2) (draft version).

Khoza, S. (2007). *Socio-economic rights in South Africa: A resource book*. Community Law Centre, University of the Western Cape.

Leclerc-Madlala, S. (2005). Popular responses to HIV/AIDS and Policy. *Journal of Southern African Studies, 31*(4), 845–56.

———. (2006). "We will eat when I get the grant": Negotiating AIDS, poverty and antiretroviral treatment in South Africa. *African Journal of AIDS Research, 5*(3), 14–20."Letter from the president," (2007). ANC Today, http://www.anc.org.za/ancdocs/anctoday/2007/at29.htm (accessed January 10, 2008).

Link, B., & J. Phelan (2001). Conceptualising Stigma. *Annual Review of Sociology, 27*, 363–85.

Macklin, R. (2004). "Ethics and equity in access to HIV treatment": Pro-poor health policy team 3 by 5, Geneva, WHO.

———. (2006). No shortage of dilemmas: Comment on they call it "patient selection" in Khayelitsha *Cambridge Quarterly of Health Care Ethics, 15*, 313–21.

Mann, J., & Tarantola, D. (1998). Responding to HIV/AIDS: A historical perspective. *Health and Human Rights, 2*(4).

"Mayor slammed for abuse of power," (2007). *Citizen*, February 28.

Mattes, R. (2003). *Healthy Democracies? The potential impact of AIDS on democracy in Southern Africa*. Occasional Paper 71. University of Cape Town.

Mbali, M. (2004). AIDS discourses and the South African State. *Transformations, 54*, 104–22.

———. (2005). The treatment action campaign and the history of rights-based, patient-driven HIV/AIDS activism in South Africa. In Jones, P., & K. Stokke, pp. 213–43.

McCoy, D. (2003). Health sector responses to HIV/AIDS and treatment access in Southern Africa: Addressing equity. Equinet discussion paper, no. 10.

McGregor, L. (2005). *Khabzela: The life and times of a South African*. Jacana Media.

Minister of Health v TAC. (2002). Constitutional Court of South Africa, Case CCT 8/02.

Mokaba, P. (2002). *The Sunday Independent* (June 16, 2002).

Nattrass, N. (2004). *The moral economy of AIDS in South Africa*. Cambridge University Press.

Nobel peace laureate claims HIV deliberately created. (2004), http://www.abc.net.au/news/newsitems/200410/s1216687.htm. (accessed January 15, 2005).

North West Mirror (2005). "Imbizo get an earful of Temba woes," January.

Norwegian Ministry of Foreign Affairs. (2002). *Fighting poverty: The Norwegian government's action plan for combating poverty in the south towards 2015. Oslo*: Ministry of Foreign Affairs.

Ntuli, A. (n.d.). Provincial findings in preparation for the South African human rights commission public enquiry into the right to have access to health care services, synthesis report.

Open Democracy Advice Centre Annual Report (2005). Annual Report, http://www.opendemocracy.org.za/documents/AnnualReport2005.doc (accessed January 11, 2006).

Palmary, I., & Ngubeni, K. (2000). "We are living in a forgotten place": Safety in the cross-border parts of the city of Tshwane. Centre for the Study of Violence and Reconciliation.

Parkhurst, J. O. (2001). The crisis of AIDS and the politics of response: The case of Uganda. *International Relations, 15*(6), 69–87.

———. (2002). The Ugandan success story? Evidence and claims of HIV-1 prevention. *Lancet 360*, 78–80.

Parkhurst, J. O., & Lush, L. (2004). The political environment of HIV: Lessons from a comparison of Uganda and South Africa. *Social Science & Medicine, 59*, 1913–24.

Patterson, A. (2006). *The Politics of AIDS*. Boulder, CO: Lynne Rienner.

Peires, J. (1992). The implosion of Transkei and Ciskei. *African Affairs 91*, 365–87.

Piot, P. (2008, May). AIDS exceptionalism. Lecture, London School of Economics.

Pisani, E. (2008). *The wisdom of whores: Sex, lies and AIDS prevention*. Granta.

Plusnews. (2005). South Africa: Rollout bogs down, http://www.plusnews.org (accessed June 10, 2006).

———. (2005). Lazarus drug: ARVs in the treatment era, http://www.IRINnews.org (accessed September 10, 2005).

Posel, D. (2005). Sex, death, and the fate of the nation: Reflections on the politicization of sexuality in post-apartheid South Africa. *Africa*, 75(2), 125–53.

Posel, D., Kahn, K., & Walker, L. (2007). Living with death in a time of AIDS: A rural South African case study. *Scandinavian Journal of Public Health, 35*(69), 138–46.

Putzel, J. (2003a). *Institutionalising an emergency response: HIV/AIDS and governance in Uganda and Senegal*. Report submitted to Department for International Development. London School of Economics and Political Science.

———. (2003b). The politics of action on AIDS: A case study of Uganda. *Public Administration and Development, 24*, 19–30.

Robins, S. (2004). "Long live Zackie, long live": AIDS activism, science and citizenship after apartheid. *Journal of Southern African Studies, 30*(3), 651–72.

———. (2005). From "medical miracles" to normal(ised) medicine: AIDS treatment, activism and citizenship in the UK and South Africa. *IDS Working Paper 252*, October.

Rosen, S., Fox, M., &Gill, C. (2007). Patient retention in antiretroviral therapy programs in sub-Saharan Africa: A systematic review. *PloS Medicine, 4*(10).

Rossouw, H. (2006). The 2005 annual Ruth First memorial lecture. University of Witswatersrand: Experiencing AIDS. *African Studies, 65*(2).

Schneider, H., Barron, B., & Fonn, S. (2007). The promise and the practice of transformation in South Africa's health system. In Buhlungu et al (Eds.), *State of the Nation: South Africa 2007* (pp. 289–311).

Schrimshaw, E. W., Siegel, K., & Lekas, H. (2005). Changes in attitudes toward antiviral medication: A comparison of women living with HIV/AIDS in the pre-HAART and HAART eras. *AIDS and Behaviour, 9*(3), 267–79.

Seiler, J. (Ed.). (1999). *Transforming Mangope's Bophuthatswana: Towards democracy in the North West province* (Daily Mail and Guardian, South Africa).

South African Bill of Rights, Constitution of the Republic of South Africa (1996). Act 108 of 1996, Chapter 2.

South Africa National Department of Health. (2003). Operational plan for comprehensive HIV and AIDS care, management and treatment for South Africa. Pretoria.

———. (2004). National antiretroviral treatment guidelines.

———. (2004). "HIV and AIDS and treatment," *Khomanani*, 1st ed.

———. (2008). Draft guidelines for the management of HIV & AIDS in health facilities.

Southall, R., Segar, J., & Donaldson, A. (Eds.). (1992). *Undoing independence: Regionalism and reincorporation of Transkei into South Africa*. Grahamstown: JCAS.

State and Jacob Zuma. (2006). Witswatersrand local division, Johannesburg, case no. SS321/o5, date-2006–04–04, Zuma's testimony, *15*, 929–87.

Steinberg, J. (2006). Mbeki's anxieties around AIDS have damaged national psyche. *Business Day*, http://www.businessday.co.za/articles/article.aspx?ID=BD4A310877 (accessed January 2007).

Stoller, N. (1998). *Lessons from the damned: Queers, whores, and junkies respond to AIDS*. New York: Routledge.

Sun. (2007). Classified ads, February 1.

"Time to sack health minister." (2006). *Sunday Times*, August 20.

"The awful state of the nation." (2005). *Mail and Guardian*, October 28.

Toebes, B. (2001). The right to health. In A. Eide, C. Krause, A. Rosas (Eds.), *Economic, social and cultural Rights* (pp. 169–90). Kluwer.

Treatment Action Campaign. (2006). Press release, August 15, www.tac.org.za (accessed August 15, 2006).

———. (n.d.). Affidavit. http://www.tac.org.za/Documents/Court_Cases/Rath/Defamation/TAC-Achmat-1.pdf, (accessed June 6, 2007).

———. (2007). Equal Treatment. May 22, 2007.

UNAIDS. (1996, 2006). HIV/AIDS and human rights international guidelines, revised guideline number 6. Geneva.

———. (2006). Global AIDS Report. Geneva.

———. (2003). Stepping back from the edge: The pursuit of antiretroviral therapy in Botswana, South Africa, and Uganda. Geneva.

United Nations Committee on Economic, Social and Cultural Rights. (2000). The right to the highest attainable standard of health. UN doc. E/C.11/08/2000).

———. (2000). General comment 14, substantive issues arising in the implementation of the international covenant on economic, social and cultural rights. UN doc. E/C.12/2000/4.

United Nations Economic and Social Council. (1966). International covenant on economic social and cultural rights. Entered into force January 3, 1976. 993. UNTS 3.

UNDP. (2002). *Human Development Report*. UNDP.

United Nations General Assembly. (2005). High level meeting on HIV/AIDS: Discussion paper for the round table on treatment, care and support. Undoc. A/59/CRP.4, United Nations General Assembly 59th session.

Van Der Vliet, V. (2004). South Africa divided against AIDS: A crisis of leadership. In K. D. Kauffman & D. L. Lindauer. *AIDS and South Africa. The social expression of a pandemic* (pp. 48–96). Palgrave Macmillan.

van Huyssteen, E. (2000). Other experiences of planning for reconstruction and transformation: A narrative of planning and development histories in Hammanskraal, paper presentation, http://www.gpean.org/aaps/Other%20Experiences%20of%20 Planning%20for%20R&T.pdf.

Viljoen, F., & Precious, S. (Eds.). (2007). *Human rights under threat: Four perspectives on HIV, AIDS and the law in Southern Africa*. Pretoria University Law Press.

Vincent, L. (2007). Virginity testing in South Africa: Re-traditioning the postcolony. *Culture, Health and Sexuality, 8*,(1), 17–30.

von Holdt K., & Murphy, M. (2007). Public hospitals in South Africa: Stressed institutions, disempowered management. In S. Buhlungu, J. Daniel, S. Southall, & J. Lutchman (Eds.). *State of the nation: South Africa 2007* (pp. 312–41). HSRC Press.

WHO. (2003a). A public health approach to antiretroviral treatment: Overcoming constraints. Geneva.

———. (2003b). Treating 3 million people by 2005: Making it happen. Geneva.

———. (2004a). Guidance on ethics and equitable access to HIV treatment and care. Geneva.

———. (2004b). Scaling up antiretroviral therapy in resource-limited settings: Treatment guidelines for a public health approach–2003 revision. Geneva.

WHO/UNAIDS. (2007). Towards universal access: Progress report. Geneva.

———. (2008). Towards universal access: Progress report. Geneva.

Zuberi, F., Jones, P., & Viljoen, F. (2004). HIV/AIDS stigma and Human Rights: A Localised investigation of Hammanskraal communities. Centre for the Study of AIDS, University of Pretoria.

Index

Page numbers in **bold** refer to figures, tables, and photographs.